The
Fibromyalgia
Survivor

Mark J. Pellegrino, M.D.

THE FIBROMYALGIA SURVIVOR
Anadem Publishing, Inc.
Columbus, Ohio 43214
614 • 262 • 2539
1 • 800 • 633 • 0055
World Wide Web site– http://www.anadem.com

The material in The Fibromyalgia Survivor is presented for informational purposes only. It is not meant to be a substitute for proper medical care by your doctor. You need to consult with your doctor for diagnosis and treatment.

PRINTED IN THE UNITED STATES OF AMERICA

ISBN 0-9646891-2-X

This book is dedicated to my wonderful family, Mary Ann, Maria, Dominic, and Rocco, who put up with me and my fibromyalgia and are truly fibromyalgia supporters.

Special thanks to Ann Evans for her help in reviewing the manuscript.

TABLE OF CONTENTS

INTRODUCTION

I am a fibromyalgia survivor. I have had fibromyalgia syndrome since I was a child but I was not officially diagnosed with this disorder until my mid-20s. At that time, I was in the midst of my Physical Medicine and Rehabilitation residency program when I started having persistent and pronounced pain especially in my neck and shoulders. One of my residency instructors examined me and discovered my painful tender points.

Since my diagnosis, I have strived to learn as much as I can by researching, reading, attending conferences, treating patients, and by personal experiences. I have come to appreciate how complex this condition really is, and how every individual is affected differently. Some people with fibromyalgia syndrome are hardly bothered by this condition, whereas others are incapacitated because of the pain.

One must first understand fibromyalgia before he or she can become a fibromyalgia survivor. I have learned to be a fibromyalgia survivor not from the medical journals or symposiums, but from fellow fibromyalgia sufferers who I have come to know and treat over the years.

In the past seven years, I have treated several thousand people with fibromyalgia. I have also started a fibromyalgia support group that has met once a month for the past five years. My fibromyalgia colleagues and I have tried to identify the specific problems we deal with and we have all worked together in trying to find successful solutions to these problems.

My first book on fibromyalgia, *Fibromyalgia: Managing the Pain,* was written to help individuals under-stand the basics of the syndrome and to try to begin managing the pain. *The Fibromyalgia Survivor* contains detailed strategies for successfully coping with this painful disorder.

There is more than one way to successfully treat pain. Those with fibromyalgia require individual treat-ment strategies as there is no universal single recipe that works for everyone. My simple philosophy in treat-ing fibromyalgia has always been to try to find whatever works. This includes a responsible, successful home program and a good mental outlook. This book will share some ideas and strategies that have worked for me and my patients. I hope it will help you develop some strategies so that you, too, will become a fibromyalgia survivor.

While this book contains detailed fibromyalgia treatment strategies, it is not meant to be a substitute for proper medical care by your doctor. All the contents in this book are for information purposes only. You need to consult with your doctor for specific diagnosis and treatment.

A Quick Review of the Basics

This book is written for individuals who already have a good fund of knowledge of fibromyalgia and understand the basics. I will briefly summarize the basic points in this chapter. For those of you who have not yet read the basics of fibromyalgia, I refer you to my first book, *Fibromyalgia: Managing the Pain*, published by Anadem Publishing, Inc.

Fibromyalgia is a syndrome of chronic muscle pain that is recognized as a distinct medical condition with characteristic findings. The pain involves many muscles, tendons, ligaments, bursa, and joints. Discrete areas of tenderness in specific locations called "tender points" are characteristic findings. The American College of Rheumatology criteria identify 18 body locations of which at least 11 must be present in order to make the diagnosis of fibromyalgia.

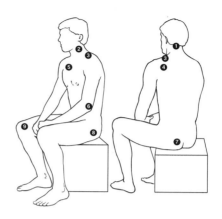

Tender points

The muscle pain fluctuates and is often aggravated by various physical, environmental and emotional factors. In addition to pain, fibromyalgia causes stiffness, fatigue, numbness, feeling of weakness, swelling, cold intolerance, poor sleep, dry eyes, as well as other symptoms. Various conditions have been linked to fibromyalgia, including tension and migraine headaches, chest pain, mitral valve prolapse, irritable bowel syndrome, TMJ dysfunction, irritable bladder, depression, and chronic fatigue syndrome.

Fibromyalgia is diagnosed more frequently in women than in men, occurring in about 2 - 5% of the population. Children can also have fibromyalgia, although the condition usually causes symptoms that begin between ages 25 and 45. Often the symptoms may be present for years even though the diagnosis may not be made until past age 50.

The exact cause of fibromyalgia is unknown, but ongoing research continues to shed light on this syndrome. There are a variety of factors that are felt to be important in causing fibromyalgia: genetics, trauma, altered neurologic mechanisms, muscle physiology problems, infectious disorders, abnormal sleep patterns, structural muscle changes, neurotransmitter abnormalities, endocrine abnormalities, immune disorders, and allergic factors. Some of the more recent research has focused on growth hormone abnormalities, abnormal biochemical mechanisms involving various enzyme systems, brain and hypothalamus disorders and altered oxygen/energy mechanisms.

After a person is diagnosed with fibromyalgia syndrome, a multi-disciplinary treatment approach often helps. It is important to educate a person on this condition, emphasizing that fibromyalgia is not a deadly or contagious disease and that a person can learn to successfully live with this condition. Various medications including muscle relaxants, sleep modifiers, anti-depressants and pain relievers can be helpful. Trigger point injections and "spray and stretch" can also help. Physical therapies, massage, manipulation, psychology, occupational therapy, and other treatments can help decrease the pain and improve one's ability to cope with this condition. A key strategy is learning a home program that works.

Fibromyalgia is a chronic and permanent condition for which there is no cure. Physicians of all specialties are learning more about fibromyalgia and are becoming better at diagnosing and treating this condition. The challenge is not only to fully understand fibromyalgia, but also to minimize its effect on the individual and the community until a cure is found.

Fibromyalgia research is moving in many positive directions, but don't wait for a cure! Get started now with your plan to become a Fibromyalgia Survivor.

Fibronomics

Trying to achieve proper posture is a well ingrained behavior of our society. We all remember the countless times we have been told to "Sit up straight" and "Don't slouch." It is as if somehow sitting properly at all times would prevent our spine from bending or curving or freezing in some abnormal position. We wondered if people with back problems got that way because they had poor posture; it was *their* fault.

We learned how to lift heavy objects using our legs and not bending over at the waist to prevent back injuries. As we became more sophisticated, we learned that there were ways to maneuver our bodies to avoid causing injuries or pain, yet still complete the functional task at hand.

The scientific study of the relationship between the human body and various tasks, particularly work tasks, is called ergonomics. Ergonomics more specifically involves designing work tasks to fit the capabilities of the human body in order to minimize the risk of injury. The human body should achieve a natural position in which there is no strain on the joints and soft tissues. The natural standing position occurs when the head is relaxed and slightly bent forward, the arms are loosely hanging down our sides with elbows bent to a 90-degree angle, the wrists straight, fingers relaxed and slightly curled and turned in, the back in a natural curve, the knees slightly bent, and the feet about 12 inches apart (see figure).

If unnatural or awkward positions occur, there is more strain on the joints or soft tissues. Examples of unnatural positions include:
• Head turned to the side or looking up
• Arms outstretched or overhead
• Elbows away from body
• Wrists bent
• Palms up
• Leaning forward
• Bending
Promoting proper posture prevents painful persons!

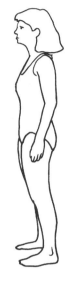

Proper posture

Those of us with fibromyalgia have a different concept of what is proper posture. All the stuff that our grandma told us just doesn't work. When we try to sit up straight for a long time, we hurt more. Slouching is actually comfortable. And, let's face it, we are not trying for modeling careers, we just want to be comfortable. Most of us who have had fibromyalgia for many years develop a characteristic fibromyalgia posture that results from countless hours in a comfortable, but less than perfect posture (see figure).

Since a different set of rules applies to fibromyalgia and posture, we need to define these rules and reprogram our minds and change our behaviors to fit these rules.

I have introduced a new term, *Fibronomics*, to define this "scientific" study of our fibromyalgia body and proper posture in our daily activities. Fibronomics can best be defined as the art of properly manipulating our fibromyalgia bodies in the environment to enable pain-free completion of a function or activity.

There are four basic rules to fibronomics. They are:

    1. **Arms stay home.**

    2. **Unload the back.**

    3. **Support always welcome.**

    4. **Be naturally shifty.**

Rule 1. Arms stay home.

Fibromyalgia muscles in the neck, shoulders and upper back areas do not like activities that involve reaching or overhead use of the arms. Isometric contractions where muscles stay contracted continuously causes decreased blood flow, decreased muscle oxygen, and increased pain. Any time the arms are away from the

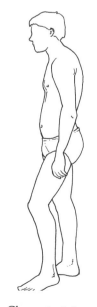

Characteristic fibromyalgia posture

body, the trapezial, scapular, shoulder and upper back muscles all go into isometric contractions which usually result in increased pain even after only a few seconds of the offending activity. Since the focus of attention is on our hands and whatever objects we are reaching for and working on, we may not notice the early discomfort signals arising out of our neck, shoulders and upper back until it is too late.

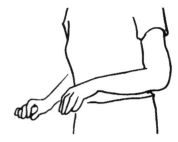

The favored position for our arms is at the sides and below the shoulder, with the elbows touching our sides and the elbows bent at a 90-degree angle (see figure). We should try to maintain this position to the point where we move our whole body, not just our arms, to confront each specific task. Arms stay home (with the rest of our body) and do not reach away.

Favored arm position

Examples of using Rule #1: Arms Stay Home

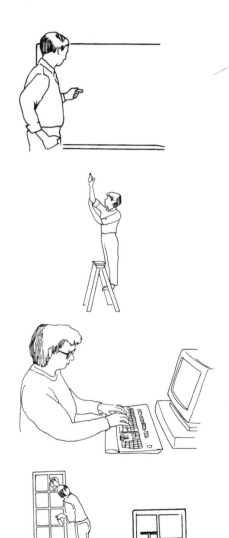

1. Problem: Reaching up to write on chalkboard
    Solutions:
      Move body closer to board
      Don't use top of board
      Use other arm to hold elbow of writing arm
      Minimize use of board, substituting some
        other visual media

2. Problem: Reaching up to change light bulb
    Solutions:
      Use stool to stand on and get closer to bulb
      Use other arm to hold "active" arm

3. Problem: Typing continuously
    Solutions:
      Chair arm rests
      Wrist bar for keyboard
      Drop keyboard mechanism
        installed in desk
      Ergonomic desk chair

4. Problem: Washing windows by reaching
      Solutions:
        Get closer to wall
        Use long handled tool such as a squeegee

5. Problem: Prolonged driving at 10:00
        and 2:00 wheel position
      Solutions:
        Use 4:00 and 8:00 positions
        Armrests
        Move seat closer to steering wheel

Rule 2. Unload the back.

The back actually includes the entire spine, pelvic and hip areas with particular emphasis on the lower back and sacroiliac regions. There are multiple internal and external pelvic and back muscles that must be equally balanced to maintain proper alignment of the low back and the pelvic areas. If anything causes a shift in this alignment, the mechanical imbalance and subsequent mis-alignment can result in a pain; pain from bones, ligaments, nerves and muscles. This is particularly true if certain muscles develop tightening or spasms and pull unequally compared to the opposite muscle. It is hard enough for our back and pelvic muscles to maintain proper balance so we need to help these muscles out whenever we can. Any activities that tend to increase the load on the back such as bending forward, prolonged standing, bending at the waist to pick up an object, or arching the back will alter the mechanical balance and increase pain.

Ways that we unload the back will avoid the offending positions in the first place. Bending forward at the waist increases the force on our back. Bending forward and reaching out with our arms causes even greater force on our back. Flexing our hip as occurs when we lift our leg and put it on a foot stool is an excellent way to unload the back when in standing position. Crossing our legs or putting our feet up on a foot rest unloads the back when we are seated. Lying in the fetal position to sleep will unload our back, and placing a pillow between the knees is especially effective at taking pressure off the hips and sacroiliac regions.

Examples of using Rule #2: Unload the Back

1. Problem: Leaning forward at kitchen sink
    Solutions:
    Back straighter, elevate leg
    Use long-handled sponges
    Open cupboard door under sink and lift leg into cupboard

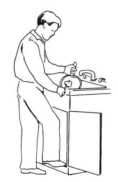

2. Problem: Riding sports bike
    Solutions:
    No ram's horn style handlebars
    Comfortable seat so back is natural

3. Problem: Carrying heavy golf clubs
    Solutions:
    Play 9 holes instead of 18
    Ride cart, pull cart or use caddy

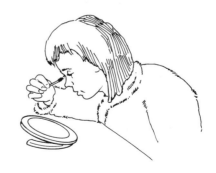

4. Problem: Applying makeup by tilting head back and
                looking into wall mirror
    Solution:
    Use magnifying mirror you look down into

5. Problem: Leaning forward at waist over a counter
                to sign papers
    Solution:
    Spread legs to lower body but maintain good back
    posture, then sign papers without bending forward

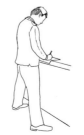

Rule 3. Support always welcome.

Whenever we can take advantage of existing structures in our environment to relieve some of the force on our bodies, we should do so. Ways that we support our back include sitting in a chair with a good seat and back, leaning against a wall or other inanimate object (and sometimes animate objects) and wearing back braces. We can support our arms on chair rests, tables, laps, our stomachs, chests (with our arms folded), on top of our head, or use one arm to support the other. Our head and neck can be supported with pillows, head-rests, neck braces, and our hands.

The days are long, and our muscles work hard to support us and get us from one place to the other. We expect our muscles to get tired, and usually before they get tired, they hurt. It is okay to use extra support to help relieve our muscles whenever we can. Our muscles won't deteriorate or atrophy if we are responsibly using additional support. We never want to reach a point where we feel we must depend on neck or back braces or other orthotics unless there is a true medical reason as indicated by your doctor.

Examples of support available:

Arms
> Armrests
> Rest arms on head, lap, or body
> Cross arms
> Hold one arm with other arm
> Furniture (table, desk, counter-top)
> Pockets, muffs, slings

Back
> Chair
> Wall
> Foot stool
> Brace, belt

Both arms and back
> Stair rails
> Pillows, cushions
> Another person's body

Rule 4. Be naturally shifty.

This rule emphasizes maintaining natural or neutral body and joint positions, but at the same time periodically moving the muscles around and shifting them. The natural or neutral positions are those that put our muscles and joints in the most relaxed physiologic position possible that minimizes unusual forces or strains on them. The basic natural body positions include: the head in a straight position with chin slightly bent forward, the low back with a natural arch or lordosis, the knees slightly bent, and the arms relaxed at the side with the elbows bent forward. We need to recognize these comfortable and natural positions, while at the same time keeping our muscles moving.

Keeping our muscles moving is one way to avoid the painful tightening and spasms that occur when we are in one position for too long. Some people have more tolerance than others but we all tend to have our limit where, if we spend too much time in one particular position, we will experience increased pain. We must learn to automatically alternate between various positions such as sitting, standing, and walking. Even within these positions we can develop strategies for shifting about to relax and stretch the various muscle groups regularly.

Our head position needs to be shifted frequently as well. This is not to be confused with our shifty brains. If we spend too much time looking up or down, or to one side or the other for long periods of time, our neck pain will increase.

Examples of Fibronomics Application

The following pages are devoted to specific examples of daily problems where proper application of fibronomics can be helpful. In each example the problem is identified, as well as the fibronomics rules that are violated, and examples of solutions are given.

1. Problem: Sitting in bleachers at a sporting event causes significant increased back pain. You want to watch your child play in a sporting event, but you cannot stand the aggravation of your back when sitting on the hard unsupported seat.

   Fibronomics rules violated:

   Rule 4) Prolonged sitting without alternating positions
   Rule 2) Sitting unsupported increases the load on the back
   Rule 3) No extra back support

   Solutions: Bring a folding chair with you to the bleachers and use it, allowing the back to be supported. Take frequent standing and walking breaks, averaging at least a minute of standing/walking for every 15 minutes sitting.

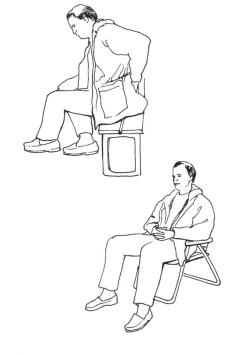
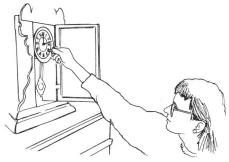

2. Problem: The clock collection is posing a problem since winding up clocks once a week causes increased neck and shoulder pain and causes arm fatigue.

   Fibronomics rule violated:

   Rule 1) Arms are reaching out to try to wind the clock, and this increases isometric contractions in the neck, shoulders and back.

   Solutions: Stand on a stool to lower the arms to a more natural position. Move closer to the clocks so the arms stay in, then wind, taking no more than 10 winds before stopping and dropping the arms down to the side for a few seconds; then resume the winding. Find a new hobby!

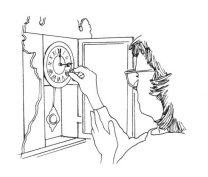

3. Problem: Getting the hair ready in the morning can cause a lot of pain, yet we have to look presentable for our day.

   Fibronomics rules violated:

   Rule 1) Arms reaching up over our head
   Rule 2) Leaning forward over the sink puts an increased load on the back
   Rule 3) Not taking advantage of any available support

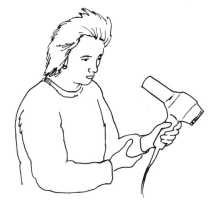

   Solutions: Use the other arm to hold the arm that is being used to fix the hair or hold the blow dryer. Hold hair dryer lower (arms more at sides) and direct air upwards. Bend head down so it is closer to the air. Obtain a folding director's type chair with a back to use to sit on in the bathroom and perform morning duties in a more favorable position. Don't be a beautician!

4. Problem: Reading and studying causes considerable increased neck pain and headache.

   Fibronomics rules violated:

   Rule 4) The sustained positioning of the head and neck causes painful tightening and increases the neck pain which subsequently leads to tension headaches.
   Rule 3) No neck support and therefore more rapid onset of neck pain because of sustained isometric contractions to maintain studying position. When studying, the focus is on the material being studied and not monitoring the early clues our neck, head and shoulders may be giving about increased pain.

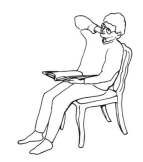

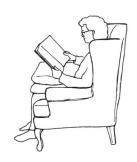

   Solutions: Alternate positions every thirty minutes from sitting at a desk to lying in bed with a pillow propped behind the head. Set a timer to remind you when it's time to change positions. Use pillow or book holder to prop up book and allow you to more comfortably adjust your head position. Lean back in chair so head and neck are more supported. Lay on bed with neck and head supported with a pillow, bend knees and put book to read on lap.

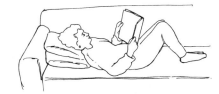

5. Problem: Sitting in a chair is painful to the lower back, and after sitting in a chair for a while and standing up, there are spasms and stiffness in the back that make it difficult to get out of a chair and stand up straight.

Fibronomics rules violated:

Rule 4) Prolonged sitting without alternating positions increases tightness and stiffness

Rule 2) Increased stress on the back

Rule 3) Failure of adequate support for the back due to poor chair design

Solutions: Crossing the legs is an excellent way to unload the back and pelvis. Remember to alternate the legs crossed. Use a footstool to rest both legs and raise the knees.

Sit in a good chair that has a sturdy back and arms to maintain proper body alignment; use a lumbar cushion or pillow to support the natural low back curvature.

When getting out of a chair, use the back peddle technique. First scoot forward to the front edge of the chair. Then plant one foot behind the chair as far as possible. With the arms pushing off the armrests, stand up while maintaining a natural back position without bending forward.

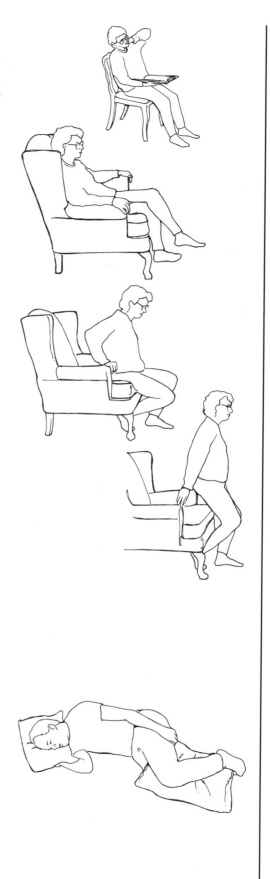

6. Problem: Sleeping on the stomach results in increased pain, awakening the person during the night and resulting in worse back and neck pain in the morning than the night before.

Fibronomics rule violated:

Rule 2) Even though one is actually sleeping the low neck and back are working hard instead of relaxing. The stomach-lying position causes back muscles to strain due to the arching that occurs as the weight of the stomach sinks into the bed.

Solution: The best way to unload the low back is to try to train yourself to sleep in the side-lying fetal position. A pillow between the knees keeps the pelvic and sacroiliac joints in proper alignment.

Make sure the pillow does not allow the head to sink too far into the bed or be pushed too far away from the bed once the comfortable position is assumed so as not to cause unnatural positioning of the head and neck.

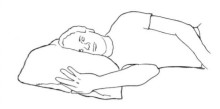

The head and neck should maintain a neutral position. Once you are in the final sleeping position, the head and neck should be aligned properly with the shoulder. In this position, individual neck muscles are not strained.

Another position that can be comfortable is lying mostly on the back, but tilting to the side with a pillow under both knees. Use plenty of pillows to pad and support the body and prevent pressure on nerves, particularly in the elbows and upper arm areas. A firm mattress with a soft mattress pad works best.

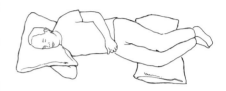

It may take a week or two to adjust to a new sleeping position, but if it is more comfortable, you will never go back to your old painful position again. Once you have trained yourself to sleep in a less painful way, your subconscious will take over and "put" you into this position during the night.

7. Problem: Getting out of bed or off the couch causes severe back pain.

Fibronomics rules violated:
   Rule 2) The back is under extreme stress when a sit-up is performed
   Rule 3) The upper body is trying to lift up unsupported before the legs swing over

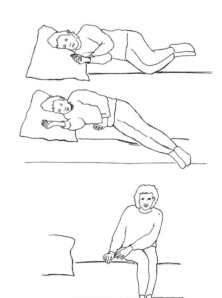

Solution: Transfer out of bed using a log roll technique. First, roll your body, log roll style, onto your side, then curl up your legs so your knees come forward and over the edge of the bed. Use the arm opposite the side on the bed to push on the surface near your waist level at the same time you swing your legs off of the edge to allow a quick yet smooth sitting up motion. This avoids undue stress on the back.

Fibronomics and specific applications will be mentioned throughout this book. You can use these rules to examine everything you do in your day. First determine why an activity may be causing pain by identifying the fibronomic rules that are violated. Don't forget those microtraumas that accumulate over time that can cause serious pain. Then analyze how these violations can be corrected and practice these new strategies until they become automatic additions to your body mechanics. You don't want the Fibropolice to ticket you for repeated violations!

Physically Managing Fibromyalgia

3

Finding a successful home program is a difficult but necessary challenge in helping us cope with fibromyalgia. It is time-consuming to treat our fibromyalgia, yet we do not want to have the pain.

There are a lot of reasons why all the muscles, tendons, ligaments and soft tissues make it difficult to stretch and exercise them. Fibromyalgia causes the muscles to be tight, ropy, and constantly in localized spasms. Our muscles do not use oxygen well and have decreased energy compounds (ATP); fatigue is a major problem.

The muscles, therefore, are painful, tight, easily fatigued, and when we attempt to exercise them they often respond by increasing pain. Negative painful experiences may lead to decreased motivation and decreased activity, or exercise phobias. A cycle of increased muscle tightness, spasms, and increased pain starts over again and we seem to sink deeper and deeper into a painful deconditioned state.

We all know the multiple benefits of a regular stretching and exercise program, yet we are also experts at knowing how much easier it is to say "exercise" than it is to actually do it. At some point each of us has to stop talking about exercise and actually start doing the exercise. Each person needs to develop his or her own home program that includes the following:

      1. Proper posture (see Chapter 2)

      2. Modalities

      3. Stretching

      4. Massage

      5. Light conditioning

      6. Relaxation exercises

Our home program is our responsibility and we have to be organized and consistent with this program. Various medical professionals can help develop a home program including your doctor (M.D., D.O., D.C.), physical therapist, massotherapist, fitness trainer, aquatics instructor, aerobics instructor, and more. As I have said over and over (and over!), no one program works best for everyone, but everyone should be able to find something that works. This chapter serves as a guideline on how to develop a successful home program.

1. Proper posture

Proper posture, ergonomics, and fibronomics are the basic building blocks of a home program. There is a proper way of doing everything in our daily lives, whether it be at home or on the job or anyplace else. Once we practice these techniques, they will become automatic and ingrained in our subconscious so we don't have to think about them all the time. These techniques are discussed in separate chapters.

2. Modalities

A modality is a physical therapeutic method of application. This includes heat, cold, electric stimulation, and water therapy. Different methods are available for delivering each modality. For example, heat could be delivered from a heating pad, a hot pack, ultrasound, or a hot whirlpool, to name a few. A hot whirlpool combines heat and water therapy. Some chemical agents can be modalities when applied to the skin to render heat or cold sensations.

From a practical home modality standpoint, heat has worked best based on my experience. Heat can be a recurrent theme throughout the day, starting with a heated mattress pad, an electric blanket, a hot morning shower, a heating pad during the day, heat-producing muscle creams before exercise, hot jetted jacuzzi after exercise, followed by a hot tub in the evening. Since many fibromyalgia patients complain of cold skin and cold extremities, heat is a natural modality to warm the skin, improve the blood flow and help relax muscles and decrease pain.

Some people complain that a jetted jacuzzi or whirlpool aggravate the tender points, particularly when there is direct pressure on them. Other people describe it as a soothing massage effect. You need to determine if this approach would work for you prior to investing in a jetted jacuzzi bathtub. A good investment for many people would be a hot tub, since it not only allows deep therapeutic heat to relax the muscles, but it is mentally relaxing as well. If a hot tub is not feasible, taking a hot bath with the water as hot as can be tolerated and soaking up to the top of your neck for 30 minutes can be an excellent substitute.

Hot showers are a great way to start off your stiff, painful morning. If you have a couple of tender areas that are particularly bothersome, a continuous hot shower stream on these areas can reduce the pain. If you are experiencing a flare-up, you can take extra showers during the day; make sure you sit in the hot tub or hot bath as well. You can never "overheat" your muscles by performing too many heat treatments during the day. This natural modality may be necessary more frequently during flare-ups, and once a stable baseline is achieved again, the usual program can be resumed.

Many people who use electric blankets will still complain of coldness coming from their mattress and sheets. I advise them to use an electric blanket only after having first acquired a heated mattress pad. Heat from below is better for skin and muscles than heat on top because the weight of our bodies pushing down on the heated surface increases the body surface area actually in contact with the heat – this improves heat conduction to the body. Plus, heat rises, so one wants heat rising from below to meet the body and not rising off and away from the body.

Some people like cold treatment. If you can stand the first 5 to 10 minutes of an ice application, then a full 20 to 30-minute treatment may provide considerable pain relief, muscle relaxation, and actually work longer than heat. However, very few people can tolerate the cold sensation against skin (including me) and opt instead for heat treatments. If heat is not effective, however, I always advise trying cold treatment whether it be an ice pack or ice massage to see if this modality is helpful.

Many people have found a TNS unit to be helpful. This is device that emits an electrical "buzz" that blocks the pain, and can be worn and used for different painful regions of the body. If this particular modality is helpful to an individual, he or she will continue to use it in spite of the hassles that are involved (putting the pads and wires in place, carrying the unit around, adjusting the controls, etc.). Some people find the TNS unit helpful, but find that the hassle involved is too great, so they choose to avoid using the TNS unit and accept the higher level of pain that occurs without using it. In the end, your home treatment has to work for you, and that means that you want to take the time to do it because the benefits outweigh the risks or hassles.

3. Stretching

Stretching is a vital part of a fibromyalgia person's home program. I consider stretching a form of exercise, and this is readily available wherever we are during our day. We need to stretch frequently during the day from morning until bedtime, and there are some helpful strategies in performing stretching exercises.

1. Always wear comfortable clothing and shoes when performing any stretching or exercises.
2. Move slowly and gently when stretching without jerking or bouncing the soft tissues. Find a feeling of stretch within your comfort zone.
3. Practice deep breathing exercises as part of stretching.

I have found that stretching exercises are the most important aspect of a fibromyalgia patient's home program. Because our muscles are so tight, they are more vulnerable to strains, so it is especially important that we counteract this tightness mechanism by stretching. I have often been asked if I had to choose one thing to do in a home program, what would I choose; and the answer is: stretching. If you are going to choose to do stretching, choose to do it regularly and consistently, stretching in the morning, stretching during the day, stretching at night, even to the point where you are stretching in your dreams! How does one begin a stretching program?

Part of my initial approach in teaching stretching as part of a home program is to train an individual in self passive stretching techniques. These do not require any specific equipment and can be done anywhere. They are very basic yet very important for increasing our muscle flexibility. Increased flexibility, in turn, leads to decreased pain and decreased vulnerability to injuries or strains.

Passive stretching exercises can be done on different body parts; head, neck, trunk, shoulder, upper body, low back, hip, and legs. Dozens of stretching exercises are possible, and all of them can be beneficial for a given individual when properly instructed. I have found a limited number of passive stretches to work very well for most patients with fibromyalgia, and the following are descriptions and diagrams of these types of self-passive stretching exercises.

Head and neck forward stretch:
Lie on your back with your knees bent and feet flat.
Place hands behind head with fingers on head and thumbs at the bottom of the skull.
Gently lift head with hands forward and chin toward chest and go to the comfort zone; hold to count of 3 to 10 seconds as tolerated.

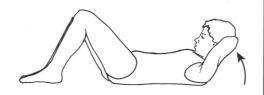

Head and neck lateral stretch:
Place one hand on opposite side of head below ear, gently pull and turn head so nose points to underarm.

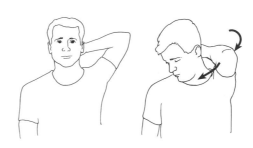

Thoracic or trunk stretches:
Cat back on all fours. Start with hands and knees on floor, head positioned between shoulders.
Let back sag, keep head parallel to floor.
Lower head with chin to chest, tighten stomach and arch back as high as possible.

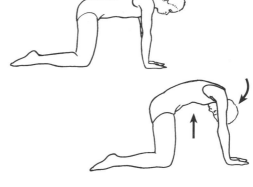

Lateral side bends:
These are performed against the wall and are called teapot exercises.
Stand up against the wall so your back and shoulders touch the wall.
Cross your arms over your head making sure that your elbows and your head touch the wall, slowly bend your upper body to your right and then to your left, keeping your feet on the floor.

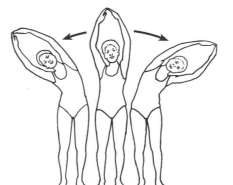

Shoulder girdle and upper body:
Hold towel overhead with hands at each end (hand towel distance), and gently pull from side to side.
Another exercise is to clasp hands behind back and lift arms upward until you feel a comfortable stretch.

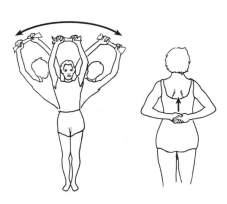
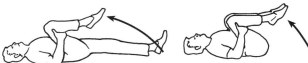

Low back:
Single knee to chest; double knee to chest.

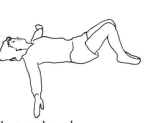
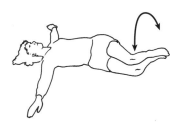

Low back and hip:
Lie on back with knees bent and feet flat on floor. Rotate knees from one side to the other.

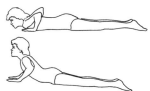

Hip flexors:
Prone push-ups; place hands under shoulders and push upper body and stop just before the stomach lifts off the ground.

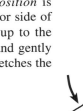

For more advanced hip flexion, the *Thomas position* is used. The individual lies on one end of the bed or side of bed with buttocks at the edge. Pull one knee up to the chest and lower the other leg towards the floor and gently bend the knee and hold as tolerated. This also stretches the quadriceps.

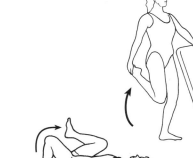

Quadriceps:
Stabilize yourself with a chair or table while in a standing position.
Pull foot up towards buttock and keep hip as straight as possible.

Hamstring stretch:
Take one knee to the chest and slowly straighten out the knee while allowing the leg to return to floor.
Hold leg as high as possible with knee straight to count of 3 to 10 seconds as tolerated.

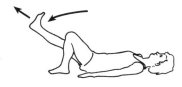

Calf: Step stretching:

Any step will work but it is best to use stairs that have a railing for better support.
Place the ball of the foot (the padding just before your toes start) on the step, letting your heel sag over the edge of the step and press down until you feel a comfortable stretch.

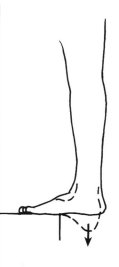

There are some general rules with stretching. Always move slowly and gently without any jerking motions, and make sure there are no restrictive clothing or jewelry. When you stretch, hold to the count of 3 to 10 seconds. When you first start off, hold for only 3 seconds, and when you become more experienced, gradually increase your ability to hold for the full 10 seconds.

Repetitions are to be started at a low number and increased. If you have been sedentary for a long period of time, you should start off with a schedule of doing all the stretching exercises only once, holding for 3 seconds with each stretch. Over the first week you progress from stretching once a day to stretching twice a day, one rep each up to 3 seconds of holding. During the second week, you progress to twice a day stretching, holding for 5 seconds, and doing 3 reps of each exercise.

For each successive week you increase the time held in each stretch by 2 seconds, and the number of reps by 2 times, until you reach a maximum of 10 seconds and 10 repetitions twice a day. (See stretch chart)

These above guidelines are particularly for a person who has been sedentary for a long while and is just beginning to start to exercise. Note that I have emphasized slow, gradual stretching over an entire month before even adding any type of conditioning type exercise. It is very important to establish muscle stretching and flexibility in a sedentary individual as part of the initial exercise program prior to performing more conditioning type exercises. One should expect the pain to increase at first when reactivating the muscles. A controlled gradual increasing stretching program as described will hopefully minimize the pain and still allow progressive improvement. Ice after stretching, muscle creams, and over the counter anti-inflammatory medicines can be used to help "smooth over" the transition period of increased pain.

Certainly one can speed up the progression process and perform various versions of stretching numerous times during the day. I recommend stretching at least twice a day in the training process, but as the individual becomes more experienced, I advise essentially unlimited stretching during the day. In fact I encourage people to always think about stretching as part of their routine day.

Passive stretching should start in bed before getting up in the morning. The following are suggested bed stretches.

Bed Stretches

The following should be done while lying in bed prior to getting up and out of bed. Stretch and hold each position for 3 seconds.

Arm and leg reach:
Reach arms up as far as you can
Legs straight out with feet and toes pointed (ballet style)

Chin tuck:
Arms behind head, chin to chest
Place arms behind head and then push head forward so chin touches chest

Neck push back:
Neck push back into pillow, then to each side
Look up and back as far as you can, pressing head into pillow
Turn head to side pressing cheek into pillow
Repeat other side

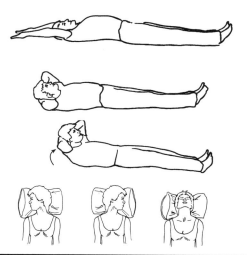

Neck extension with chin press:
Start to tilt head back; at same time try to press chin into chest

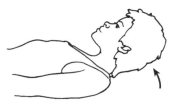

Alternate knee to chest (on back):
Bend knee to chest, holding with same side arm
Repeat other side

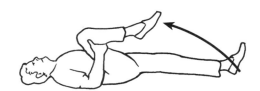

Hug self:
After stretches completed, log roll out of bed using proper body mechanics
   Good morning!

Stretching in the shower can be especially effective since you can use the warm water modality. In addition, it helps you start off your morning with stretching at a time when your muscles are usually the tightest.

These pages have given examples of stretches in different situations. One can stretch any part of the body, and I have not demonstrated every possible stretch. An excellent reference book is *Stretching* by Bob Anderson.

Exercise using elastic bands (Therabands) can combine dynamic stretching and strengthening for our muscles. These are not considered aerobic exercises, but can be very effective in increasing flexibility and strength. The rubberized elastic bands come in different colors which represent different strengths or tensions. These elastic bands may look flimsy and one may wonder how they can be effective in an exercise program. As flimsy as they look, they can provide excellent resistance for the muscles. The harder you pull and stretch them, the more the tension on the muscles. Thicker bands provide more tension.

I have found Theraband exercises to be effective in many patients. These exercises require instruction and practice to work best. Sometimes you don't realize how hard you are working with the bands, so you need to be careful not to overdo the first few times you use the bands. Once the exercises are learned, the individual can perform them as part of a self-program.

Here are some examples of basic Theraband exercises that can be helpful in stretching and strengthening the upper body and arms especially.

1. Place a towel rolled horizontally behind neck and another towel rolled vertically between the shoulder blades. Knees should be slightly bent and back flat against a wall.

   Tuck neck into the towel, roll shoulder into the wall with arms rotated outward.

   Slowly work arms up the wall. Don't forget to breathe!

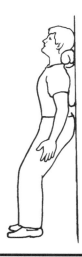

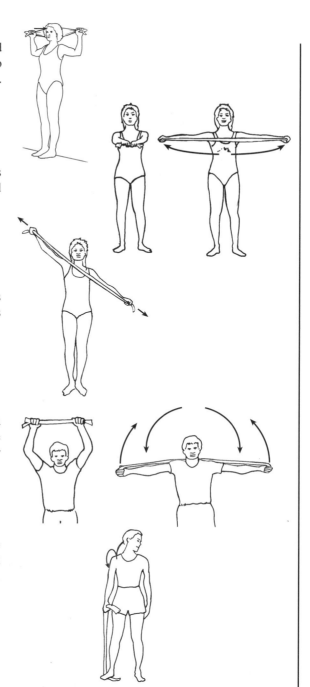

2. Place the Theraband behind head. Knees should be slightly bent and back flat. Push head into band so that chin stays parallel with the floor. Push straight back. Don't forget to breathe!

3. Take the Theraband in both hands; start with arms straight out in front and pull arms backwards until they touch the wall.

4. Take the Theraband in both hands; start with arms straight out in front of you diagonally. Pull arms backwards until they touch the wall.

5. Start with your arms overhead holding a Theraband. Pull downward until your arms are level with your shoulders. Hold your shoulder blades down as you relax your arms upwards.

6. Place a Theraband under one foot. Turn head so that the chin is over opposite shoulder and look down. Grasp the theraband and roll shoulder up, back and down without bending your wrist.

One should practice deep breathing techniques while doing these Theraband exercises. Once a person is comfortably instructed, he or she should begin a regular Theraband program ranging from 3 times a week to every day. Like stretching exercises, the Theraband should be slowly moved to position and then held to the count of 3 and slowly returned to the starting position. There is resistance from the bands during both the stretch and return. Up to 10 repetitions of each exercise can be gradually achieved for one's individual tolerance. I advise my patients to routinely perform therapy and exercises whether or not they are having pain.

One woman who had particular upper back pain learned theraband exercises that she found very effective in keeping her pain under control. However, after she stopped doing the exercises in January because of various other projects, she experienced a flare-up of her upper back pain in February. Her flare-up persisted in spite of continuing the other components of her program. Once we realized that she had stopped her theraband exercises, she resumed them and reported that her upper back pain decreased and stabilized again. This is an example of how this particular exercise can be helpful, but it needs to be continued on a regular basis. *If the exercises work, you will do them!*

Stretching Guide

	Sun	Mon	Tue	Wed	Thur	Fri	Sat
Week 1							
Reps	1	1	1	1	1	1	1
Hold	3 sec	3 sec	3 sec	3 sec	3 sec	3 sec	3 sec
Times Daily	twice	once	once	once	once	twice	twice
Week 2							
Reps	3	1	1	1	2	2	3
Hold	3-5 sec	3-5 sec	3-5 sec	3 sec	3 sec	3 sec	3-5 sec
Times Daily	twice	twice	twice	twice	twice	twice	twice
Week 3							
Reps	5	5	5	5	5	5	5
Hold	5-7 sec	5-7 sec	5-7 sec	5-7 sec	5-7 sec	5-7 sec	5-7 sec
Times Daily	twice	twice	twice	twice	twice	twice	twice
Week 4							
Reps	7	7	7	7	7	7	7
Hold	7-9 sec	7-9 sec	7-9 sec	7-9 sec	7-9 sec	7-9 sec	7-9 sec
Times Daily	twice	twice	twice	twice	twice	twice	twice
Week 5							
Reps	9	9	9	9	9	9	9
Hold	5-10 sec	5-10 sec	5-10 sec	5-10 sec	5-10 sec	5-10 sec	5-10 sec
Times Daily	twice	twice	twice	twice	twice	twice	twice
Week 6							
Reps	10	10	10	10	10	10	10
Hold	5-10 sec	5-10 sec	5-10 sec	5-10 sec	5-10 sec	5-10 sec	5-10 sec
Times Daily	2 or more as needed	2 or more as needed	2 or more as needed	2 or more as needed	2 or more as needed	2 or more as needed	2 or more as needed

Reps: the number of times each stretch is done
Hold: how many seconds each stretch is held
Times Daily: how often a day the stretching is done

4. Massage

Massages are a wonderful way to decrease pain, relax muscles, improve blood circulation, passively stretch muscles, and overall feel good. Massage is probably one of the oldest pain remedies; there have been written records of massage from over three thousand years ago by the Chinese.

There are definite physiologic effects of massage. These include reflex effects which are produced in the skin by stimulation of nerve receptors. These nerve receptors cause relaxation of muscles and increased blood flow, resulting in a sedative effect.

There are also mechanical effects of massage which include improved flow of blood and lymph, and muscular motion which stretches muscle fibers and increases flexibility. Massage does not develop muscle strength and therefore is not a substitute for active exercise, but mechanically it produces effects that actually simulate passive exercise.

Massage is a combination of art and science. There are multiple effective styles of massage depending on the individual's natural ability. The personality of the therapist is just as important in deriving positive benefits as the actual massage skill of the therapist.

When choosing a massotherapist, I think it is important that you do your homework. Make sure the therapist is licensed and is knowledgeable and experienced in treating fibromyalgia. You don't want to feel that your therapist knows very little about your problem since this will interfere with your potential benefits from the treatment. Patients have the best luck when they choose massotherapists based on word of mouth from other fibromyalgia patients.

There are several basic techniques used in massage. Stroking (effleurage) is performed by running the hand lightly over the surface of the skin. This may be superficial or deep and it assists in the blood and lymph circulation.

Compression (petrissage) includes kneading, squeezing, and friction. Kneading and squeezing involves grabbing the muscles between the palms and fingers or between the thumb and fingers, and working the muscles as if kneading dough. A slow and rhythmic motion works best. Squeezing is performed with larger portions of the muscle, either between the two hands or the hand and a solid object such as a table. Friction is a circular type motion performed by placing a small part of the hand, usually the thumb or fingertips on the skin and doing circular loops with increasing pressure.

Percussion (tapotement) are alternating hacking movements usually done with the outside of the hand, and alternating movements as if playing the drum. Clapping is a similar technique only done with the palms of the hand.

The various techniques of massage are not done one after the other, but are intermingled, and different techniques are used for different purposes. Each massotherapist has his or her own style and personality. Certain specialized forms of massage such as myofascial stretch and release and trigger point pressure therapy can be incorporated as part of an overall massotherapy technique.

My patients, as a rule, have found traditional massotherapy techniques to be most effective on their fibromyalgia muscles. When a massotherapist experienced with fibromyalgia performs a massotherapy on a patient, the universal response is one of decreased pain and relaxation, which may last for hours or days, or longer. Massotherapy can be incorporated into part of an overall treatment program and may often be the best technique for an ongoing supportive and maintenance program.

Massotherapy could be done daily if a person had access to this treatment. However, our health care system does not allow the personal delivery of such daily intensive treatment, so I usually recommend an approach of once a week to start for a period of 6 to 10 weeks, then 2 treatments a month for several months, and then, if feasible, 1 to 2 treatments a month on an ongoing basis.

It has been my experience that massotherapy is not aggravating to the muscles, even though we are very sensitive to touch and pressure on our skin. The first 1 or 2 treatments can often cause increased muscle soreness, so using ice, heat, creams or medicines afterwards may be needed. Once the muscles become used to the technique, the usual response is one of considerable relaxation and decreased pain. Usually people will leave the massotherapy room with a natural euphoric feeling.

There are numerous devices on the market that give a mechanical massage. Many people find these devices helpful especially when performing self-massage techniques, but this is never a substitute for a "real" massage by a trained therapist.

Self-massage is a fairly simple procedure that can be learned and performed effectively. Individuals can learn to perform various techniques such as compression and stroking on themselves. Family members or significant others can also be trained to perform therapeutic massages on the fibromyalgia patient.

Self-massage is a common helpful technique, especially if there are painful knots or tender points in "reachable" areas. Long-handled devices are available for those "unreachable" areas. Self-massage can be performed any time during the day but is often best done in the shower where the hand can glide easily by using soap. Stretching can be combined easily with self-massage. One massotherapist who has worked with hundreds of fibromyalgia patients likes to instruct patients on giving themselves a hug when taking a morning shower. This allows stretching, self-massage, and starts the day off with a hug!

5. Light Conditioning

People with fibromyalgia usually do not tolerate a lot of exercise, as a general rule, but a little bit of exercise is helpful. A light conditioning program means enough exercise to stimulate the cardiovascular system and strengthen the muscles without overworking or exhausting them and causing increased pain. Various studies have shown that exercise is good for fibromyalgia and remains one of the best treatments.

Realistic goals need to be set for the body that is well beyond high school! We have to realize what we can reasonably accomplish, i.e., be able to perform a good workout 30 minutes, 3 times a week. Don't put pressure on yourself that you have to exercise longer and harder in order to feel better. I always tell patients that the amount of time spent exercising is not as important as the actual effort to exercise.

A light conditioning program should not be started until an individual is comfortable with a regular daily stretching program. If one has been sedentary with fibromyalgia for a while, then stretching exercises alone should be done for a full month before attempting any light conditioning program. For individuals with fibromyalgia who are more active, a light conditioning program can be started soon after a regular instruction program has been achieved. Light conditioning exercises should be performed at least 3 times a week for 20 to 30 minutes. As a rule, one should take off every other day with a light conditioning exercise program to allow the body a chance to rest and recuperate, but different individuals can perform a daily exercise program depending on their own body's abilities and needs. When starting out, it is best to perform about 10 minutes per session for the first week, and then gradually increase 5 to 10 minutes per week until at least 30 minutes 3 times a week is reached. Remember not to let our overachieving bodies do too much.

Light conditioning does not necessarily entail intensive aerobic activity for 30 minutes. Often the activity itself involves periods of stretching, strengthening, relaxation, and actual conditioning. This alternating strategy usually works best for our fibromyalgia muscles which do not like too much of one thing at any given time. Doing any conditioning program involves proper warm-up, breathing techniques, good posture, awareness of body's response to the program, and a cool-down period. Various forms of exercises could fall into this category of "light conditioning" and include weights, walking, cycling, stair machines, arm pulleys, aquatics, aerobics and dancing.

Weight-lifting is a category of exercise that emphasizes strengthening, but there are some stretching and conditioning components as well, if higher number of repetitions are done. People with more severe forms of fibromyalgia usually do not tolerate any type of weight-lifting whether it is free weights or machines. It appears that the continuous resistance on the muscles over-stimulates the muscles and increases the pain.

For individuals who have tried weight-lifting and continue to experience increased pain, I usually recommend avoiding weights altogether. These people should use alternative exercises that allow more variable resistance on the muscles, which is usually tolerated better. Many people with milder forms of fibromyalgia can develop a very successful weight-lifting program without the muscle flare-ups. In these people, the goal should be lesser weight and more repetitions to minimize microscopic tears or strains to the muscles, and increase their endurance and energy. Free weights and variable resistance weight machines seem to work best. If your fibromyalgia has reached a point where you have a difficult time doing any type of exercise, I would not advise attempting a weight-lifting program on your own. If you participate in a supervised therapy program in which weights are introduced and tolerated, then you may incorporate this into your home program. In simple English, we are not the type to join a health spa and try to exercise like everyone else!

Walking can be a very effective form of light conditioning exercise. Natural walking should be done while wearing soft cushioned comfortable shoes, such as tennis shoes. Rubberized tracks are the best surfaces to walk on as they minimize the impact to your feet and ultimately your back. Walking with a buddy, who can be your spouse or friend, is a great way to motivate and commit yourself to this type of exercise.

When first beginning a walking program, you can alternate 5 minutes of brisk walking with 5 minutes of more leisurely walking, and repeat this cycle. The goal is to gradually increase your brisk walking to at least 20 to 30 minutes 3 times a week.

Some people do not tolerate walking because of particular pain in the low back, hip or leg areas. However, others who have predominantly upper body pain may find walking the best way to loosen up these sore muscles. The upper body and arms also get involved with walking, particularly brisk walking with a lot of arm swinging. Increased heart rate and stimulated respiratory drive makes this exercise a beneficial cardiovascular and aerobic activity as well.

Many people prefer to use a treadmill for controlled walking exercise. I thought I would enjoy this type of activity, but after I purchased a treadmill, I found this type of walking to be too artificial. There is something about walking but not seeing things move around you that bothers me. I have a hard time maintaining an exact rhythm as I prefer to be able to vary my pace and I tend to lose my balance every so often. I found that a slight loss of balance on the treadmill could throw me off the treadmill entirely! Even though I prefer natural walking, I still encourage people to consider treadmill walking if they are interested, but try it first before you purchase the machine. If you like your trial, I know where you can get a cheap treadmill that has hardly been used!

I am frequently asked if any certain exercise equipment is helpful in fibromyalgia. I always advise people that anything can be tried, but before making a large purchase, one should try several sessions of exercise on that particular piece of equipment, either at a health spa or at a friend's house. If you determine you like the exercise, and you tolerate it well and feel it is helpful, then you can consider purchasing it. Too many of my patients have exercise equipment sitting in their basement that has hardly been used.

Here are some considerations for different types of exercise equipment:

Exercise cycle:
The biggest potential problem is malpositioning on the unit. If the seat is too narrow, or the handlebars are too far out in front, you could be in a position where you are leaning forward and reaching out with your arms. This can create a lot of neck and back strain. Wide, comfortable seat and handlebars that reach out to you so you can hold them and still be in a comfortably aligned position are necessary. Persons with painful knees may not tolerate stationary bikes at all, but the seat height can be adjusted higher to decrease the strain and painful movements on the knees. Exercise cycles that allow a reclined position can be very effective for fibromyalgia patients since these minimize the strain on the low back and arms.

Stair machine (Stairmaster):

This equipment emphasizes strengthening the gluteal and leg muscles. Many people with fibromyalgia can only handle this type of machine for a short period of time before there is increased cramping type pain especially in the calves. Those with knee pain may find this exercise too aggravating to their knees. If you can tolerate and progress with this machine, it is an excellent workout.

Arm pulley systems:

These systems may be part of a treadmill, stationary bicycle, or other leg exercise apparatus. The main problem with this type of system, in people with fibromyalgia, is that it puts a lot of strain on the arms, particularly with all the reaching, pulling, and squeezing involved. The arms usually tire very quickly. People who have difficulty reaching out with their arms will usually not tolerate any arm pulley system as part of their exercise program, but some systems don't require as much "reaching" and can be tolerated well.

Another popular form of exercise is aquatics. Water exercises provide an opportunity to stretch, strengthen, and condition the body. The water supports the spine and extremities and acts as a brace and massager. Those who have difficulty holding their arms out in front may do so more comfortably as the water buoys the arms. Standing chest high in water will remove much of the gravity in the lower back area, which may dramatically reduce pain.

Numerous aquatic exercise classes are available for people with arthritis and fibromyalgia. Warm water is necessary. Ideally the water temperature should be 87 degrees or higher, although many pools keep the temperature for these types of classes around 85 degrees. Various aquatic equipment is available to help individuals work out in the water.

Like other forms of exercise, one needs to first try the water program to determine if it is helpful. Some individuals do not tolerate the cold feeling in the water or the air drafts that can occur and cool the skin. Wearing a wet suit or long sleeve shirt in the pool, and having lots of dry towels ready as soon as you exit the pool can help avoid the cold feeling.

Others describe the process of changing into a bathing suit, getting into the pool, getting out of the pool, showering, drying the hair, and getting dressed again to be too much of a hassle even though there may be some benefits. However, many people, particularly those who have tried land exercises without success, and who may have particular problems with their low back, pelvic, hips and leg areas, respond very nicely to an aquatics exercise program. I recommend that these exercises be done first with an aquatics instructor, usually in a group-type class. Choose a pool with warm water and warm, still air around it! Individual programs can be developed if group aquatic exercises are helpful.

Traditional aerobics are not tolerated very well by people with fibromyalgia, since it involves a lot of exercises with the arms out or overhead, prolonged standing, and high impact on the body. Low impact aerobics may be better tolerated. The arm exercises and standing are still difficult for many people. Step aerobics are popular and some individuals with milder fibromyalgia may do well with this type.

Modified aerobics, if tailored to the fibromyalgia individual, can be an effective light conditioning exercise program. I have worked with an aerobics instructor in my area to develop "chair aerobics," particularly for people with fibromyalgia.

Chair aerobics involve following fibronomics. The individual is seated as much as possible to unload the spine. Activities are done primarily from the chest level and below, avoiding any arm overhead activities. Movement exercises are still performed but instead of higher impact movements, there is a modification. For example, walking movements may be simulated by having the individual "march" while seated in the chair.

Stretching is emphasized and the problem areas are moved slowly. The exercises are designed to stretch the tight muscles, usually the chest and quadriceps, while strengthening the weaker muscles, usually back and hamstrings, and to try to achieve a better posture. Therabands are commonly used in chair aerobics.

Many fibromyalgia patients who participate in group chair aerobics indicate they are more comfortable with this approach since they are working with people who have the same problem. This type of class can function as a support group.

Even though the group of people works together in a class setting, the program is flexible enough that individuals can do their own techniques within the group format. The individuals are encouraged to follow through with these exercises on their own at home. If they enjoy the program, they will continue with the class setting once a week as well.

Many of my patients have found dancing to be a great workout for them that is tolerated well. Jazzercise, line dancing, polka dancing and good old rock and roll dancing are examples of light conditioning and aerobic exercises that have worked for various people. Some like to dance to video tapes and others will get out to public dance floors. Remember to stretch and warm up before turning yourself loose!

There are numerous types of exercises that can be done. The key, as always, is to actually do something. Professional guidance and supervision are available to help you find a program that is right for you but it is your responsibility to do something, and do it regularly and consistently. You should stretch before and after exercising, and you should stretch just about any other time in between! You may prefer to exercise at home because you can be more independent and flexible with your program in a convenient location. You also don't have to worry about being embarrassed by others watching you, if that is a concern.

On the other hand, working out in a gym or spa allow you to get away on a predictable schedule and be in a social setting. Paying for a membership often motivates a person to follow through regularly, and positive results will increase your confidence and self esteem.

Activation of muscles can be painful at first, but it is not harmful to the muscles. You are not hurting yourself and you will be able to "work through" this initial pain.

Temporary flare-ups can occur when one is starting an exercise program, but support and supervision from your medical professionals when starting your rehabilitation program will enable you to overcome any initial difficulties and get "over the hump," so to speak.

Once a successful exercise program is underway, I believe that subsequent flare-ups are very rarely due to the actual exercise program. Rather, the flare-ups are due to some other cause (see Chapter 7 on flare-ups). However, you may need to modify your exercise program during the flare-up. It is important that you continue your exercise program in spite of the flare-up. You may need to reduce or modify the exercise program, especially for the flared-up muscles. If you stop using or exercising muscles that were flared-up, these muscles will get tighter and will quickly become "deconditioned;" that is, they will get weaker and have less stamina. Once you're deconditioned, it becomes even harder to reactivate the muscles. Thus the "curse" is that muscles that are flared-up still need to be exercised to keep them as flexible and conditioned as possible, even though they hurt more. Adding extra modalities can also help relieve your flare-up to return to a stable baseline. Don't stop everything, though. You will be surprised that you can still follow through with an exercise program even if you have more pain.

Mentally Managing Fibromyalgia

4

We all know that the mind has influence on the body and it is a powerful healing tool. Mental stresses can literally create illness and diseases of the physical body. Likewise, physical conditions causing pain or disability can influence the mind and create problems such as depression, anxiety and negative thinking. The mind and the body are both affected in fibromyalgia.

Physically fibromyalgia causes pain, fatigue, weakness and dozens of other symptoms. Mentally it causes depressed mood, mental fatigue, poor concentration, anxiety, and dozens of other symptoms. This chapter is devoted to strategies to manage the mental aspects of fibromyalgia. It is possible to use the mind to help the healing process in fibromyalgia. Note that healing is not the same as curing. Curing implies permanently alleviating a condition, that is, completely getting rid of fibromyalgia. Healing, on the other hand, implies going through a process of restoring and improving health and well-being even if the condition is not eliminated.

Stress is a major factor in our fibromyalgia. Although stress does not cause fibromyalgia, it certainly aggravates it. Life is synonymous with stress, however, so we can never get rid of stress. We can learn how to reduce stress and minimize how it bothers our fibromyalgia.

There have been hundreds of articles and books written on how to reduce stress, relax and think positive. Do all of these strategies work? In general, yes they can. Do they work for everyone? No, but many people can definitely benefit from mental techniques to manage their physical problems. There is no one "right" way, as there are many ways that can work. The trick is to get the individual to attempt any way. It takes a lot of motivation, practice, and perseverance to successfully learn a mental management strategy, and not everyone is able to do this. Some patients are not able to go through this alone and may need a professional counselor to assist them.

The reason that it is so difficult is that we have gone through life learning to define a certain set of rules, and thought processes, and have applied them to our individual situations. Through the years we have evolved a very specialized thought process on how we view ourselves and our world. Then all of a sudden, fibromyalgia comes along and these rules and processes no longer effectively apply. We are then asked to change our lifestyle, not only physically, but mentally. This is not an impossible task, but it involves a willingness to try to take that first step and make a commitment to change our lifestyle. It is natural to be scared or even terrified of this process. But with encouragement, patients with fibromyalgia are truly impressive in their ability to face this difficult issue and achieve a positive mental outlook.

How can one make mental lifestyle changes? I try to approach this in a series of smaller steps, steps you build upon and integrate together to accomplish a big leap into a new successful mental approach to managing fibromyalgia. I also try to keep things as simple and organized as possible. I have devised a mental strategy which I call the **5 "REpairs"**:

1) **RE**cognize and **RE**define

2) **RE**alistic **RE**training

3) **RE**liable **RE**lationships

4) **RE**lax and **RE**fresh

5) **RE**spect and **RE**sponsibility

Each "pair" is intimately related and addresses a different aspect of the mental approach to fibromyalgia. The ultimate goal is to be able to integrate all 5 "REpairs" into a positive mental strategy that works best for you.

1. REcognize and REdefine

As a rule, we think negatively with fibromyalgia. We first need to recognize the ways that we think negatively, or ask "What do we think?"

Ways we think negatively

a. Leap from one thing to over-generalization. For example, if we forget something or are forgetful, we think we are getting Alzheimer's disease.

b. We anticipate bad things. For example, if someone invites us to a party, the first thing we think of is that the party will cause a flare-up in our pain.

c. We blame ourselves for everything. We believe it is our fault that we have fibromyalgia or that we have flare-ups.

d. We label ourselves negatively. We tend to think that because we are having a lot of pain, we must be bad or useless people.

e. We expect things to get worse. For example, if we are talking to someone older than us who has fibromyalgia and is having extreme pain and disability, we expect that we will end up like that person when we get older.

We need to recognize that continuous negative thinking about ourselves and our situation will ultimately lead to various negative emotions such as anger, frustration, hopelessness, and feelings of guilt and depression. Many of us have developed a low self-esteem and feeling of worthlessness.

We should also recognize that we tend to be perfectionistic and over-achieving individuals, and this can lead to negative consequences when trying to cope with fibromyalgia. Our perfectionistic nature can create "negative" traits which include:

- Inability to handle criticism
- Fear of failure
- Fear of rejection
- Inadequacy
- Anxiety
- Lack of control

By being overachievers, we also risk developing negative consequences which include:

- Always searching for a fibromyalgia cure
- Doctor shopping for that magical treatment
- Inability to delegate tasks to others
- Feelings of being overwhelmed
- Procrastination
- Impatience
- Extreme guilt when unable to accomplish what we used to be able to do

We must recognize the ways that we think negatively, and how some of our innate personality traits can create negative consequences in the presence of fibromyalgia. This recognition is necessary for us to progress to the next step, to redefine our thinking patterns.

To redefine, we ask ourselves, "What goals do we wish for ourselves?" and "How do we want to see ourselves?" and "What can we do?"

Fibromyalgia forces us to redefine our physical ability. Since we can no longer do what we used to be able to do, we must seek a new physical lifestyle that our fibromyalgia allows us to tolerate. We also have to redefine our thought processes. We must now think of ourselves as persons with chronic pain, and from that perspective, try to imagine how we can feel better about ourselves.

A part of redefining our thinking is to try to redefine what it means to feel good. Since we are so focused on feeling bad all the time, it is hard to look for things about ourselves that make us feel good.

You certainly must stop blaming yourself for your fibromyalgia. You were not singled out to have this painful disorder for something you did or did not do! Fibromyalgia is very common, and you know that you are not alone with it. Tell yourself you are a good, normal person who happens to have fibromyalgia, and work on believing it. Expect to live a life of good quality in spite of having fibromyalgia.

For our personality tendencies of being perfectionistic and overachieving, we should try to redefine those qualities and see the positive instead of the negative. Examples of positive outcomes of our perfectionistic tendency include:

- Organization and efficiency
- Industriousness
- Responsibility
- Trustworthiness
- Reliability
- Punctuality

Being overachievers can also have positive consequences which include:

- Innovative thinking that allows us to create new strategies
- Being an active participant in our care and decisions regarding fibromyalgia
- Reading everything we can about fibromyalgia and therefore acquiring a very good knowledge
- Learning to budget our energy and break big tasks into smaller tasks

Ultimately, we need to recognize that fibromyalgia is a chronic illness. We need to take an inventory of all of the thoughts we have and how we feel about ourselves because of fibromyalgia. We then sort through this inventory to determine what we want to throw out, modify, change -- what we want to redefine. We are smart and we are ready to put our knowledge to good use. The next step in the process is realistic retraining.

2. REalistic REtraining

At this step, we ask the question, "How will we change our thinking?" With fibromyalgia, it is not realistic to expect to be pain free. However, it is realistic to achieve a low baseline level of pain where we feel we are able to enjoy our lives as fully as possible.

Retraining our thinking is not an easy or quick process. It took us a long time to reach where we are in our thinking process, so it will take time to change our thinking as well. A "quick fix" is not a good strategy since it only captures our initial enthusiasm and motivation similar to some of the fad diets. We need a slow but long-lasting lifestyle change that has a higher chance of being successful for a longer duration.

A lot of people have been trained to think in black and white; it is either one way or the other. If we are then forced to look at different shades, to start exploring the gray areas, this can create a lot of tension and even confusion in some people. However, we already have a condition that is not in the black and white area. That is, fibromyalgia is not normal, yet it is not a disease. It is nestled in that gray area and we need to allow ourselves to look into and explore these mental gray areas. You may be surprised at the new mental strategies you can learn in that territory.

Part of retraining the thinking process is to follow through on what you recognize to be the negative parts of the thinking process, and shift the focus to positive. We've read everywhere about the benefits of positive thinking. I try to encourage my patients to recognize that they can affect the outcome of their fibromyalgia in a positive manner. No one has to end up like someone they've talked to who also has this condition.

The individual with fibromyalgia who makes the effort has a much better chance of positively affecting the outcome than the person who does nothing to start the adjustment or acceptance process. Some of the studies done on fibromyalgia patients over time have found some fascinating comparisons: Individuals who took an aggressive role in seeking strategies to control their fibromyalgia are less bothered by fibromyalgia as they get older. Those who took a passive role or were never given the opportunity to become an active participant in the management of the disorder fared much worse.

Retraining yourself to think more positively is certainly a challenge. I think it is best that guidelines are given, but that each individual seek his or her own technique.

Like setting physical limits, you need to set mental limits as well, and learn to accept these limits. You must allow yourself at times to be forgetful about things, but not let it convince you that you have a memory disease. You can allow yourself to be critical of your performance, but don't punish yourself personally, and feel that you are worthless, or unable to do anything. You can worry about certain activities causing a flare-up, but you have to set a limit on this. You can't let it cause you to become inactive and avoid any type of activity.

Try to train yourself to stop thinking "I shouldn't" and change it to "I'll try." That way, instead of completely avoiding, or mentally turning off the thought of a certain activity, you force yourself to look at that activity and try to find ways to complete the activity, whether partially or completely. Try to find gaps in this "wall" blocking the activity that you can break through and get to the inside. This is a way of thinking positively, yet still remain within your mental limits. This also forces you to think of strategies and mentally rehearse these strategies as a positive and constructive way of approaching your perceived problems and limitations from fibromyalgia.

If you can train your mind to look for that opening and rehearse a way to get through that opening, the physical aspect will follow a lot easier. An example of this approach is as follows: a minister with fibromyalgia experiences a severe flare-up following a flu syndrome. Because of increased pain and fatigue, she is no longer able to perform her weekly hour-long Sunday service that includes a 20-minute sermon. She thinks that she shouldn't even try to complete a Sunday service because of too much preparation required, not to mention the prolonged standing and hand gestures that she prefers while giving her sermon. Her initial thought is to avoid the Sunday service altogether until her flare-up resolves and she is able to perform all of her usual duties.

However, because of the uncertainty of when her flare-up would resolve, and because of the importance of her involvement in the church, she takes a new approach. She re-examines every activity she does during her Sunday sermon and tries to find ways to participate in these activities. She mentally perceives a plan in which she would first perform only the sermon, the vital part of the overall service. She would do this activity from a seated position and minimize the hand gestures, and shorten the service from 20 minutes to 10 minutes. From this she envisions being present during the whole service but being seated in a chair. Over the course of several Sundays, she would gradually increase her own participation in the service as tolerated. She rehearses these mental strategies and constructs her plan, and then physically carries this out. She finds out that she is still able to enjoy the important Sunday activities as an active participant in spite of her fibromyalgia flare-up.

A retraining process does not work 100 percent when you first try it, and a successful behavior is never 100 percent perfect. Before we learned to walk, we first had to balance ourselves, learn to stand, learn to take slow, deliberate and unsteady steps, practice this pattern until it became easier and more automatic. Finally we developed our walking skills that became part of our subconscious physical ability. We had to fall down many times at first before we became proficient at walking and even though we can walk well now, we still fall down every so often. Our walking skills were achieved by a series of small, successful steps that were inefficient at first, but with practice, gradually became a successful and efficient system, although not 100 percent perfect. This is also how our mental retraining process works.

Mental retraining strategies can make physical performance easier. But doing physical things can also help us mentally feel better. If we make an effort to physically look well (dressing nicely, keeping our hair neatly styled, basic good grooming), we will feel better about ourselves, and thus receive a mental boost. Proper diet, achieving ideal body weight, and following through with a regular exercise program are also ways that make us feel better, both physically and mentally.

3. REliable RElationships

This REpair step involves others in your life.

Relationship means family, spouses, significant others, friends, and co-workers. Your fibromyalgia not only affects you, but all those around you. Relationships change because of fibromyalgia, and often times they can change for the worse. It is your responsibility to make your relationships positive in spite of fibromyalgia.

Even though you are in constant pain, your goal is to treat the ones you care about with compassion and kindness no matter how bad you feel. This isn't easy because you hurt and feel downright mean and miserable. You might find yourself being short tempered and unpleasant with the ones you care about. You can feel very guilty about these situations. You are allowed to feel miserable and be mean and short tempered. You can have these feelings or moods and still be a good person! You simply recognize that these are negative consequences of your chronic pain and you are going to work hard on overcoming these even if you aren't perfect at it.

There is also the tendency to shut out the family and caring ones because of your pain. Essentially you shut out the world because of your pain. Instead of the pain being less, the pain is actually noticed more because the world around you has shrunk so small that there is nothing else in it except you and your pain.

Don't shut out your relationships. Keep them in your world. Let your family help you and allow yourself to play an active role in educating and communicating with your family.

Many times, families and significant others do not know how to respond to you and your fibromyalgia. If you do not communicate your problems, your family will not be aware of them. They may play a guessing game to figure out how you are feeling at any particular time.

Some families and patients react to a chronically painful problem by denying the existence of the problem. They think that your fibromyalgia is something that will simply go away some day and you will be back to your "normal" self. You need to educate your family and significant others on what fibromyalgia is all about. Give them literature to read. Let them know how they can help you. Let them know what types of things aggravate your pain, what you are doing to help control your symptoms and what works for you. Tell them that your fibromyalgia is not a tumor and will not cause deformities or paralysis and that you will not die from it. Hopefully, they will appreciate your teaching attempts.

Communicate openly with your family and others you trust. You are not the only one who has frustrations, needs and feelings about the fibromyalgia; they do too. Share your feelings with them, find out their feelings, and work together to understand and accept your limitations, both physically and mentally. Work on positively redefining relationships.

In relationships, everyone brings his or her own unique perspective. Each person's perspective has been shaped by his or her individual past experiences, traumas, attitudes, limitations, accomplishments and much more. Everyone has "baggage." Most of our baggage, however, just happens to be from our physical experiences with fibromyalgia. Just as we would not reject someone for something in their past, we would not expect someone else to reject us just because we have fibromyalgia and a "past" associated with this problem. If we give others a chance, they can accept us.

You will still have bad days, and your family is still going to have bad days. At times you will think that no one is making any attempt to understand your problem, and at times they will think that you are simply using fibromyalgia as an excuse to avoid your responsibilities. A successful family support system is one that recognizes the extremes that occur occasionally, but maintains a stable balance of understanding, acceptance and support that does not falter when these occasional bad times occur. Family life (indeed, any relationship) is difficult even in "normal" situations. Adding a chronic illness to the situation makes everything even more challenging.

How can a family or individuals work together to form positive and reliable relationships? Open communications is important. It helps if your family reads about fibromyalgia and maybe even attends your fibromyalgia support group. Have frequent family conferences that function as your own family support group. Find out how everyone is feeling and how family members can help each other out. If you find the problem is too big to handle on your own, you may wish to seek professional help.

It is difficult for fibromyalgia people to ask others for help. Our feelings of low self-esteem, fear of losing our independence, and concern that we will be bothering this person by asking for help inhibit us. However, fibromyalgia prevents us from doing the things that we want to do and it is important for us to learn to ask for help and to delegate responsibility of various tasks to others.

As a family, team chores can be performed by different family members who have a designated task as part of a bigger chore. Everyone works together and performs his or her task. The fibromyalgia person also participates in the chore by performing the task that he or she is able to do.

One patient compared this process to a corporation. If you are the CEO of the family, you have the ultimate role of making sure your whole family unit is functioning. However, you can set up your organization so problem solving and simple task completion can be done at different levels. Not everything has to go directly to you, the CEO, to be handled. Even though you are ultimately overseeing everything and involved with everything, you don't need to be approached directly for every task or problem. With your influence, these tasks are already being automatically handled.

It is okay to ask for help from others. We need to allow ourselves to approach reliable and trusted individuals and ask for help when we need it. Instead of "bothering" these people, we will probably discover that this person will gladly help us and will feel good about being able to help us. Family, friends and co-workers can become trusted people who we could learn to feel comfortable communicating with, and asking for help. One patient of mine said that whenever she is feeling her lowest, she always calls her most positive friend and can count on her to boost her spirits. We all need to find these positive people that can help pick us up when we are feeling down.

An area of concern to many patients with fibromyalgia is sex and intimacy. Chronic pain and illness definitely impact this aspect of relationships. There are particular fears and anxieties on whether individuals will be able to find an accepting life partner, or continue to have satisfying and fulfilling relationships once chronic pain and fibromyalgia have intervened.

Open communication between the partners is certainly the most important factor in dealing with sex and intimacy problems. Partners need to discuss what hurts or what helps. For example, certain positions may be painful for a partner with fibromyalgia, but other positions are not. Educating a non-fibromyalgia partner on things that help such as hugs, massage, and things to avoid such as back slapping and squeezing tender points is necessary.

The doctor's role is to review concerns and provide suggestions. It is important to reassure the fibromyalgia patient and partner that the fibromyalgia does not physiologically interfere with the sexual functions. However, certain medications (particularly the anti-depressant medicines in the selective serotonin reuptake inhibitor family) can cause sexual dysfunctions. I have a particular patient who took one of these medications and felt it helped her fibromyalgia and depression very well, almost miraculously, but it interfered with her ability to achieve orgasm. This was particularly distressing for her because her intimacy with her partner was one of the only things she was able to enjoy in spite of her fibromyalgia. In situations like this, the doctor's role is to try different treatment and medication options with the patient to seek a balance between improving fibromyalgia and minimizing interference with sexual function.

Many patients benefit from professional counseling with a health professional who is experienced in treating problems related to sex and intimacy. Both the patient and partner are involved with this therapy. Individuals will often benefit from talking to other individuals with similar problems, sharing ideas and providing support.

Support groups are an excellent way to form reliable relationships. Sharing with others who know exactly how you feel has incredible power. Many of my patients are active in computer Internet where they participate in a computer interactive fibromyalgia support group. Volunteering to help others is an excellent way to stop thinking about our own problems and feel good about helping others deal with their problems.

4. RElax and REfresh

Perhaps one of the hardest things for people with fibromyalgia to do is to relax. With fibromyalgia we always seem to have tense bodies and minds. One woman described her tense mind as though she is "constantly running a marathon in her brain." We have a more hypersensitive autonomic nervous system, especially the sympathetic nervous system which is responsible for the "fight or flight" response.

The "fight or flight" response is triggered when we are in a threatening situation. Certain hormones, especially adrenalin, are released in large quantities to ready the body's protective mechanism, and we become tense, focused, and are primed to either fight or run. It is not often though that a tiger jumps out of a bush in a parking lot and starts running after us, nor do we usually find ourselves standing in the middle of a railroad track facing an oncoming train. Yet somehow we manage to maintain a continuous state of anxiety and tension in our lives and seem to be in a constant low-grade "fight or flight" mode. Imbalances of various brain hormones may occur (i.e., norepinephrine, serotonin, dopamine) which result in "mental" symptoms such as difficulty concentrating, forgetfulness, mental exhaustion and irritability.

The relaxation response is the opposite of the "fight or flight" response. The relaxation response occurs when natural physiologic mechanisms cause muscles to loosen up, blood flow to improve, heart rate to slow down, and mind to become calm. This response is chemically mediated by our body's parasympathetic nervous system and it often becomes eliminated or distorted when the body is in a constant state of tension and anxiety.

If we have lost the ability to subconsciously achieve the relaxation response, we need to consciously retrain our bodies to relax again.

If there ever was a time when something was easier said than done, it has to be telling someone with fibromyalgia to "relax." It is so difficult to "relax" that whenever someone tells me to relax, I actually get more tense. Paradoxically, saying the word "relax" actually elicits a fight or flight response! When trying to teach yourself a relaxation response that works best for you, keep in mind that there are literally dozens of ways that one can learn to relax, and, as I have said before, there is no one way that works best for everyone, but there is probably one way that would work best for anyone.

Whether one is meditating, preparing to play a sporting event, praying, or performing tai chi, a type of relaxation exercise is being mastered. You too can learn to master the art of relaxation.

The first rule of relaxation is to establish a comfortable environment. This means picking a quiet spot and turning off any noise, making sure that there are no phones to disturb you. Find a comfortable chair where you can stay in the same position for 20 minutes without increased pain. To get yourself comfortable, make sure you wear loose, nonrestrictive clothing, place your body in a neutral position, then close your eyes.

The next step to the relaxation response is deep breathing. Once you have achieved your comfortable position and have told your muscles to relax, you should become aware of how you are breathing, and if you are breathing properly. Your stomach moves out when you breathe in through your nose and contracts in as you slowly breath out through your mouth.

Take slow deep breaths through your nose and take in as much air as your lungs will hold to the count of 3. When exhaling, breathe out slowly through a slightly opened mouth to the count of 6. Placing your hands on your stomach will give you tactile feedback that your stomach is properly moving out and in as it is supposed to with deep breathing. Repeat this cycle for 10 to 15 minutes, then sit quietly for 5 minutes with eyes either open or closed, continuing to think only calm thoughts.

Do not be disappointed if you don't achieve a deep trance or hypnotic state. This rarely happens. Breathing deeply can make you feel dizzy or lightheaded at first. Try to stay relaxed as you feel yourself about to pass out! This exercise should be done at least once a day, but can be done several times a day if necessary.

The relaxation response is the most basic relaxation exercise and can be an important part of your fibromyalgia management, once you practice and master this technique. There are other types of relaxation exercises, many that involve mental imagery. Daydreaming, fantasizing, and recalling pleasant memories are examples of mental imagery that can help to relax. This type of technique can be done while you are performing other activities, and can be done with your eyes open. Many people can perfect this technique and induce a form of self-hypnosis which helps achieve successful relaxation.

Biofeedback can help individuals to learn to relax. This technique is performed by trained psychologists or counselors, and involves muscle monitors and skin temperature measuring devices. Small surface electrodes are placed on the various tight muscles and the individual can learn to relax muscles by reducing the "noise" of the muscle tension. Likewise, the skin temperature monitors can be placed on the hand or certain part of the body and the individual can learn to warm up the body part, which is a physiologic consequence of achieving the relaxation response (blood vessels to the skin will dilate and thus the skin temperature will elevate). Depending on the biofeedback instructor, it is my experience that biofeedback is successful in 50% to 60% of people. Success means the ability to learn how to relax and carry this same response over into your everyday life.

The following are examples of ways people can achieve relaxation in their lives and to help them cope with fibromyalgia.

a. A regular exercise program: This is a powerful stimulator of the body's relaxation response.

b. Religion and prayer: Many people are comforted by their beliefs and convictions in a better place than their painful existence on earth.

c. Taking up enjoyable hobbies.

d. Volunteering to help others.

e. Taking a hot bath or enjoying a hot tub: This is a great way to both physically relax the muscles, and mentally relax the mind.

f. Writing: Keep a daily journal or diary; write a fibromyalgia survivor book!

g. Music: A universal stress antidote.

h. Taking drives on a rural freeway or country road during the day. (Avoid the construction or slow semi-trailers in front of you!)

i. Playing video games, particularly the hand-held type: My favorite is Tetris.

j. Spend 15 minutes a day looking at 3-dimensional pictures; this is actually a great exercise to divert your thoughts and relax your mind and body.

Relaxation is not something that just happens. It is something that you first practice, and in time accomplish a successful technique. Then you must plan your relaxation response on a daily basis. Set time aside and protect it for yourself. This is not the time to take a nap, but an opportunity to manage your fibromyalgia.

5. REspect and REsponsibility

The final step in repairing your mental approach to fibromyalgia is Respect and Responsibility. Having a painful syndrome is difficult because every day you hurt, and I know this from personal and professional experience. We must understand and respect that fibromyalgia indeed does cause pain, lifestyle altering pain, and that we will continue to have pain. If your goal is to completely eliminate pain, you will be setting yourself up for disappointment because that is an unrealistic expectation. Rather, set a goal to achieve a minimal baseline level of pain. Try not to avoid doing something for fear of flaring-up your fibromyalgia; rather do whatever you can in spite of your fibromyalgia and its pain. You remember how you used to be before fibromyalgia, but now it is time to re-set your mental thermostat to a level that accommodates some baseline pain.

The issue of control and fibromyalgia comes up frequently. I have taken the approach that fibromyalgia is a condition that we have no control over; we either have fibromyalgia or we don't.

However, we can learn to appreciate and respect the control we do have once we have the condition. We are able to control our posture, our response to stress, our activities, our home program, etc. We focus on respecting what we can control so we can decrease the risk of a fibromyalgia flare-up. In spite of doing everything right, however, we will still experience fibromyalgia flare-up whether it be idiopathic, or related to weather changes or other uncontrollable elements. Even though we have no control over these flare-ups, by taking care of what we can control, we will still have fewer flare-ups overall than if we did nothing at all.

I use the concept of good vs. bad pain as part of the control issue in fibromyalgia. If we have control over certain activities that we choose to do, we can deal with the consequences of increased pain, if this pain is expected. If we want to wash the car one warm Sunday, then we can choose to wash the car and accept the increased pain we experience on Monday (and Tuesday, Wednesday and Thursday!) because we performed an activity we wanted to do, and because we want a clean, shiny car. On the other hand if we choose not to wash our car on Sunday, and still wake up Monday with unexpected and severe pain, we consider this bad pain, or pain that we have no control over. The concept of controlling good pain is that we can choose to do activities we enjoy, and accept the consequences. It is better to make responsible choices despite having fibromyalgia than to use fibromyalgia as an excuse to evade responsibility.

Fibromyalgia is a part of you, but it is also a part that we want to try to get rid of. We need to seek a balance between detaching ourselves from fibromyalgia, and integrating it into our everyday lives.

We tend to detach ourselves from our fibromyalgia by trying to ignore it or pretending we don't even have it, especially when the pain level is lower. We may not follow through with our home program by rationalizing that there is no need to since we "don't have a problem."

Yet on the other hand, fibromyalgia is a very personal part of our lives that goes with us wherever we go. No matter how much we may try to ignore it, it is always there to remind us that it is part of us. I am an optimist and believe that everyone can eventually find that balance, but he or she has to work very hard at it.

Acceptance is the ultimate mental coping mechanism where we "validate" who we are. Unless we can accept ourselves, we cannot expect the rest of the world to do so, and our "official" status in the world seems questionable. I think the people who have the most difficult time dealing with fibromyalgia are those that can never truly accept it. They may know a lot about it and read everything about it, but they refuse to accept it as a condition that they truly have.

Acceptance is actually the end result of going through various mental stages and coping with a bad situation. Five classic stages of grief have been described and include denial, anger, bargaining, depression, and acceptance. Individuals progress through each stage in a chronological fashion after being faced with a serious dilemma. For example, when a person learns that he is dying of cancer and has only a certain amount of time to live, he will demonstrate typical coping behaviors (stages). These stages are as follows:

Denial: The person does not believe this is happening to him and denies that the cancer even exists. The diagnosis is simply a mistake as the doctors will soon realize.

Anger: This is the "Why me?" stage. A person asks "How could I get this? What have I done to deserve this?" and is very angry at the world.

Bargaining: The person is beginning to feel more hopeless and desperate. He promises to be a better person if only this cancer would be cured.

Depression: The person realizes that the cancer is incurable and goes through a period of clinical depression.

Acceptance: The person finally accepts his incurable disease and prepares for the end. He tries to appreciate the quality of the life that he has left.

These five stages are also experienced with death of a loved one or debilitating diseases (for example, spinal cord injuries, stroke, rheumatoid arthritis).

With fibromyalgia, it appears that individuals have a harder time progressing through these stages. They often move back and forth among the various stages, and may never reach the acceptance stage. I believe this is because fibromyalgia is not as predictable as other incurable conditions such as cancer. With predictable conditions, there is usually a defined pattern or course that the disease will take, with an anticipated end point. With fibromyalgia, there is no way to predict what will happen, when a flare-up will occur, or how a person will be twenty years from now. Consequently it is difficult to progress through various stages.

What can often occur is that a patient with fibromyalgia displays denial, anger, bargaining, and depression at different stages. If the condition is relatively stable, there may be a return to denial because the person finds it to be the best mental coping mechanism. "I'm feeling better, therefore I must not have a problem anymore." Once a flare-up occurs, however, the person may return to anger, bargaining, and depression. This bouncing around in various stages makes it difficult to reach the final stage – acceptance.

People can get caught up in this cycle and start feeling desperate and panicky. Doctor and therapist shopping, compulsive shopping, eating binges and other types of behaviors are common when people get caught up in these confusing cycles. We need to realize this and be warned that this is the time when we are vulnerable and may try any therapy at any price. Professionals may help in resolving these cycles and achieving acceptance of this chronic disorder.

Because acceptance is such an elusive "prize" to many people who are trying to mentally manage their fibromyalgia, I think that once this level is truly reached, it is most appreciated and people will stay at this "stage."

Achieving acceptance provides you with a powerful mental tool necessary to manage fibromyalgia and reintegrate into your world with fibromyalgia. You need to see yourself as making a positive contribution to your community, being an important and valuable part of your circle of family and friends, and overall having a positive quality of life. Modifying your work in order to remain gainfully employed, volunteering at a hospital, getting out with your friends on a regular basis, participating in family chores, and exercising and stretching on a daily basis are all active ways that you can enjoy the highest quality of life in spite of having fibromyalgia. You know that there are no miracles in terms of a fibromyalgia cure, or magic medication at this time. But you can have hope that you will be able to live the type of life that you want in spite of fibromyalgia, and hope that our research will result in a cure someday.

Fatigue and Fibromyalgia

5

Fatigue is a major complaint in people with fibromyalgia in addition to the muscle pain. Chronic fatigue syndrome (CFS) is a condition which many physicians feel is very similar to fibromyalgia. In fact many medical professionals feel that the two "names" are actually the same condition. Chronic fatigue syndrome may be a subset of a broader fibromyalgia syndrome. Both fibromyalgia and chronic fatigue syndrome can be precipitated by a viral infection, physical illness, or a trauma.

Persons with chronic fatigue syndrome have a major criteria of chronic fatigue causing at least 50% reduction in overall activity for six months. The person with chronic fatigue syndrome also has other associated conditions including sleep disorder, headache, muscle pain, joint pain, abdominal pain and recurrent sore throat. Doesn't this sound like fibromyalgia?

In chronic fatigue syndrome and fibromyalgia support groups, both pain and fatigue are frequent topics of discussion. These problems are described as the worst ones. Overall, I treat patients with chronic fatigue syndrome the same way I treat patients with fibromyalgia.

Fatigue is actually a combination of physical and mental factors. The correct definition of the word fatigue is a physical state of discomfort and decreased efficiency from prolonged and excessive exertion causing loss of power and capacity to respond to stimulation. This definition implies that fatigue is a normal consequence of prolonged or excessive physical stress on normal muscles. Fibromyalgia muscles do not require much before they become physically fatigued. In fact, our muscles become tired and exhausted rather easily.

This muscle fatiguability may be predictable. That is, we can identify certain activities or times of the day when our muscles always feel fatigued. Many people report late in the afternoon as the time when the muscles start to wear down. Those who work at a job that requires a lot of standing and walking will likely experience leg fatigue, whereas those who do a lot of assembly line work requiring repetitive use of the arms will complain of arm fatigue. The increased fatigue is closely linked to the increased pain.

In additional to usual activities, "unusual" activities can cause fatigue. Going shopping at the mall, playing a game of basketball, and walking up several flights of steps are examples of activities which can bring about sudden increased fatigue in the muscles.

One steel worker once described his leg fatigue occurring at the end of the workday as turning him into a Slow-Mo camera. He felt like his legs were working in super slow-motion with each move being highlighted and requiring detailed concentration. (He is a die-hard football fan, by the way!)

Unpredictable fatigue is common with fibromyalgia. It is often much more frustrating because it can strike the muscles without any precipitating activity. The muscles suddenly feel very lazy and can't get started. Another person described her fatigue as a feeling of driving along and idling at a stop light when suddenly the car runs out of gas and stalls. (She is not an auto mechanic, by the way!)

Extreme fatigue has a mental component as well as a physical one. Neurasthenia is a medical term that describes the extreme lack of energy and feeling of exhaustion as a result of mental factors. This mental fatigue makes it hard for one to concentrate or focus on a task because there seems to be no mental energy or ability to think sharply.

Here is an example of how a patient describes her mental fatigue. "I feel like my mind is in a fog and it doesn't want to make the connection to tell my body what to do. It seems like I have to motivate myself and talk to my arms and legs to get them to work, otherwise they won't want to do anything. I feel like I want to go to sleep."

Why do patients with fibromyalgia (and chronic fatigue syndrome) have such a problem with fatigue? There are probably multiple reasons and a combination of factors that cause and contribute to fatigue in fibromyalgia. These reasons include:

1. **Non-restorative sleep disorder.** By not getting good quality sleep, we are not accomplishing restorative events that should be occurring during the deep stage of sleep. Our bodies do not manufacture proteins and replenish energy stores as efficiently when deep sleep is lacking.

2. **Deconditioned muscles.** Deconditioned muscles in fibromyalgia have decreased ability to make the body's energy molecules called ATP (adenosine triphosphate). This energy molecule is stored in our tissues, particularly muscles, and is used as fuel to enable our body to perform all of its functions, including muscle contractions. The less ATP around, the less energy available, and once the stored supplies are used up, fatigue occurs. If this process occurs quickly, one may feel a sudden, unpredictable energy crash.

3. **Constant pain.** The body's process of monitoring pain, recording pain, and expressing pain is an energy-consuming process that involves nerves, neuro-transmitters, and other various enzymes and hormones. The patient in constant pain will use up more energy and have less stored than a person without constant pain.

4. **Decreased oxygen use by the muscles.** Studies have shown that muscles with fibromyalgia do not use oxygen as well as normal muscles. This may reflect a problem with the mitochondria in the muscles, the small organelles that use oxygen and manufacture ATP. There may be a biochemical problem or inefficiency that prevents the available oxygen from being used efficiently and adequately to create ATP.

5. **Associated clinical depression.** Depression is seen in many patients (nearly half) with fibromyalgia and can cause extreme mental fatigue.

6. **Associated chronic conditions** such as arthritis, hypothyroidism, or other disease. People with fibromyalgia and other conditions may have excessive fatigue from both the fibromyalgia and the energy consumptions of these other chronic conditions. Hypothyroidism causes fatigue due to the lack of thyroid which is a common hormone responsible for helping produce energy in the body. People with anemia have a lack of red blood cells to gather and transport oxygen. Arthritis and other conditions cause pain and inflammation which consume energy.

7. **Cognitive factors**. There is an inherent "neurasthenia" factor with fibromyalgia that causes difficulty with concentration and attention, increased anxiety, increased sensitivity to depression, and absent-mindedness.

8. **Hypersensitive autonomic nervous system.** We are more prone to anxiety and panic attacks, Raynaud's phenomenon, fast heart rate (especially in response to stress), rashes on the skin (especially in response to touch), throat tightness, and other symptoms that are all consequences of an oversensitized autonomic nervous system. The autonomic nerves are the small nerves in the body that interconnect the major nerves with the various tissues such as blood vessels, bones, muscles and organs. These nerves are responsible for keeping the internal body in harmony with the outside environment. Examples of body functions that are managed by the autonomic nerves include sweating, digestion, pain regulation, blushing, and more. The hypersensitivity of this neurologic system probably demands and depletes more energy, thus less is available for muscle activity and movement.

9. **Visual hypersensitivity.** I use this term to describe the difficulty we have whenever we are in grocery stores or department stores, or trying to negotiate a myriad of signs while driving. We try to spot on a particular object but are confronted with a variety of shapes, sizes, colors in different directions that literally overwhelm our visual senses and at times cause a feeling of dizziness, lightheadedness and increased anxiety. This is probably a combination of cognitive factors, and a hypersensitive nervous system, but I believe this contributes to fatigue.

10. **Decreased respiratory endurance.** Many patients with fibromyalgia complain about their inability to perform short bursts of activities such as climbing steps, running or walking swiftly without feeling extremely short of breath and actually having difficulty "catching their breath." This respiratory complaint may be from sudden fatigue of the respiratory muscles which disrupts the breathing rhythm in response to exercise.

    This complaint seems to be independent of whether or not the person is deconditioned or living a sedentary lifestyle. Since an efficient breathing process is necessary to deliver oxygen into our bloodstreams, any problem in this area will certainly create potential for fatigue.

11. **Constant muscle movements.** People with fibromyalgia are frequently shifting their bodies to find more comfortable positions. Habitual movements such as tapping fingers on the table, tapping or bouncing the feet on the ground, frequent crossing of the legs, and kicking out of the leg are probably subconscious movements to relieve muscle stress, keep the blood flowing, and readjust the muscles and posture to try to decrease the pain. However, the side effect of these types of movement patterns is increased energy consumption.

12. **Hormonal problems.** Growth hormone and thyroid hormone have been found to be low in people with fibromyalgia. These hormones are important in regulating the body's metabolism. Lower production of these hormones, or inefficient use of the available hormones can be a factor in the fatigue. Other hormones that may be involved include estrogen and cortisol. Serotonin, a brain hormone, has been found to be low in fibromyalgia which probably causes mental fatigue.

Whatever the cause of fatigue, it creates problems in our daily activities. The major "bad" effect of fatigue is increased pain which in turn consumes more energy and causes further fatigue. This creates a negative self-perpetuating cycle of pain and fatigue.

Fatigue interferes with our ability and motivation to socialize, carry out daily routine, necessary chores, and perform our job properly. When one is fatigued it is difficult to converse or communicate, thus interfering with our relationships. Muscles become more de-conditioned and we experience decreased overall cardiovascular fitness. We may develop feelings of depression and overall decreased well-being. Even if we have no energy, we still tend to feel stressed and, like the pain, the additional stress consumes more energy and further increases our fatigue.

There are some strategies for treating fatigue. Fatigue will probably never be eliminated, but there are many things that can be done to control its consequences and minimize its impact on everyday life. Your doctor may first want to investigate for underlying diseases such as hypothyroidism, anemia, and connective tissue disease, which involve different treatment approaches. If there are no significant underlying diseases present, the fatigue may be attributed to part of the fibromyalgia syndrome or chronic fatigue syndrome.

What steps can be taken to minimize the potential debilitating effects of fatigue? Below is a list of strategies which I have found helpful:

1. **Develop good sleep habits.** Quality sleep is necessary to enable the body to manufacture energy. Develop a good sleep routine where your body gets trained to recognize a certain time of the evening along with a certain series of events indicating "sleep time." A sleep routine may include the following: No caffeine after supper, a hot bath, relaxation activity such as reading, listening to music or watching TV, writing a list of things to do the next day and then "clearing the mind," going to bed at the same time each night, and sleeping in a comfortable position. Your doctor may prescribe a sleep modifier to help achieve a better quality sleep.

2. **Avoid daytime naps.** Although fatigue may be compelling at times, it is best to try to avoid taking naps during the day since this alters the body's sleep rhythm. Naps are often non-refreshing and time-consuming. Upon awakening from the nap, many people report feeling even less energetic and more difficulty getting going again. They may even have a period of increased confusion and mental fogginess.

In some people, however, a strategic nap accomplishes its goals in refreshing and restoring the individual to enable more successful completion of the rest of the day. As long as the evening and primary sleep is not disturbed, these naps are not to be discouraged. However it is my experience (and sleep studies show) that most people who try to nap to overcome fatigue actually do not accomplish the refreshing and restoring mood that they are seeking, and the evening sleep pattern becomes more disrupted.

3. **Proper nutrition.** Certain dietary foods can increase fatigue. Diets especially rich in fat can put the body into a lazy mode. Many of my patients have found that reducing their fatty intake has caused increased energy.

4. **Medications, natural and prescription.** There are dozens of natural vitamin supplements in foods that have been advertised as increasing energy. (see chapter on Alternative Medicine) Some people report positive results with increased feeling of energy when trying these products. Many energy products contain caffeine or ephedrine which act as stimulants and can have long-term adverse effects on the body. Before trying any natural energy product, I recommend first consulting with your doctor.

Certain prescription medicines can be prescribed by your doctor in cases of extreme fatigue causing debilitating daily problems. These medicines are the same ones used for children with attention deficit disorders. If underlying depression is a problem, your physician may opt to prescribe an anti-depressant medication because improving the depression will usually improve the fatigue as well.

5. **Follow proper fibronomics.** Maintaining proper body posture at home and at work will not only preserve energy, but decrease pain.

6. **Planned scheduled activities, especially in the evening.** The late afternoon and early evening are often the most difficult times for persons with fatigue. After supper can be an especially difficult time and if the person sits down to relax or lies down to read the paper, this is often followed by "crashing" with extreme fatigue and inability to perform any useful activity for the rest of the evening.

My advice is to routinely plan some activity, especially after supper, that may include running errands, getting outside, visiting people, or just staying up on your feet and doing something. You will be surprised to learn how frequently a "second wind" will come. Many people's biorhythm have low energy in the late afternoon and early evening, but then the mood and energy level swings back up again. If you are a night owl, you know that you tend to start feeling better and more energetic around 9 PM and may have a few good hours where you feel alert and can accomplish a lot. Recognize your own biorhythm and take advantage of it to plan your best work around your high points and to try to stimulate yourself through the low points by involving yourself in an activity.

7. **Divide your task into smaller projects instead of one big project.** Do a little at a time and do more at your best time. For example, yard work can be divided into specific chores for different nights of the week. The front lawn may be mowed one night, the back another, and the trimming can be done on a third night, instead of all three of these activities in one day. A good example of breaking up a big project into small tasks occurs when we become self home movers. If we are moving and decide to do our own packing, it is much easier to pack a box per day for the six weeks prior to the actual moving date, than to try to do all the packing one or two days before the actual move. This type of self-discipline is also needed when vacationing and decorating for the holidays.

8. **Perform regular exercise and relaxation.** Exercise increases endurance, cardiovascular conditioning, and a feeling of well being. Relaxation decreases stress and reduces pain. Taking a 30-minute brisk walk after supper can accomplish exercise, mental relaxation, and working through the low biorhythm point at the same time. It really is possible to both mentally relax and physically exercise at the same time! One does not have to be sitting down perfectly still to physically and mentally relax; in fact, this often increases the fatigue and tendency to sleep. Remember to relax, not nap.

9. **Make a daily schedule and check off things as you accomplish.** Allow plenty of time to complete the task. By keeping a structured list, you have a better chance of motivating yourself to accomplish your established daily goals.

10. **Delegate chores to others.** One of the best energy-saving techniques known is to have someone else use his or her energy to accomplish your task. While delegating responsibilities is difficult for many people, there are others who will gladly perform certain chores for you or assist you in doing the more energy-consuming portions of that chore. It is best to be as independent as possible, but it is better to allow someone else to help if it means you will have more energy to be more independent for a longer portion of your day.

Hopefully some of these "weapons" can help you combat your fatigue. Remember that fatigue, like pain, is a "relative" problem. That means that the problem is always there, but you try to achieve a lower, more functional state that, relative to the previous level, is considered a successful, manageable level. (It doesn't mean your relatives have a problem!)

Alternative Medicine and the Treatment of Fibromyalgia | 6

In the past few years, there has been an increasing awareness of alternative medicine strategies to address the needs of patients with fibromyalgia. The practice of medicine is often divided into conventional or traditional approaches, and alternative approaches. Persons with chronic pain problems such as fibromyalgia have found that a blend between these two practices of medicine often works best for managing the condition.

Conventional or traditional medicine emphasizes the diagnosis and pharmacologic treatment of various medical conditions based on scientific research. The main philosophy is identifying the cause of disease, and treating it with medicines or surgeries to eliminate the cause. Conventional medicine cures the patients with bacterial infections by treating them with antibiotics, rescues the individual with acute appendicitis by performing an appendectomy, saves the person with diseased organs by performing transplants, controls diabetes by providing insulin shots and countless other examples.

However, conventional medicine often fails the patient with chronic pain who does not respond to medications or is not a candidate for a surgical procedure. Furthermore, people with chronic pain problems, especially fibromyalgia, often undergo countless, expensive diagnostic tests including laboratory studies and specialized x-rays and electrical testing which usually do not result in any specific diagnosis. This can be very frustrating for the patient who is told that nothing was found after undergoing all of these various tests.

Conventional medicine sets the standard for scientific studies. If a certain study shows a particular drug to be effective in the treatment of a disease, for example, this study gives scientific validity to the use of this particular drug for the disease. Scientific studies are a valuable tool in proving effectiveness of certain treatments, or if a particular treatment is harmful to individuals. Scientific studies ultimately help and protect the patients.

Scientific standards can be a double-edged sword sometimes. For example, the patient's report of "feeling better" from a certain treatment usually cannot be scientifically measured. Therefore, a particular treatment may be reported to be extremely effective, but if there is no scientific research to support this, the "scientific standard" cannot be met and thus the treatment is not given any scientific credibility.

The placebo effect has a built-in negative connotation in conventional medicine and scientific research. A placebo is something that "pleases" an individual, or, from a medical standpoint, causes the individual to report improvement in symptoms even though the actual treatment did not cause any measurable body responses. A person who reports improvement in his pain after being given a sugar pill is said to have had a placebo response to the sugar pill. No measurable body responses would be obtained when giving a person a sugar pill. In scientific research, the placebo response would refer to how people respond when they are given a sugar pill instead of the drug being tested. The placebo in conventional medicine is undesired, because it is a human response to hopefulness and wanting to get better with a treatment. Thus, the placebo response needs to be "cancelled out" in scientific studies. However, the positive response to hopefulness and desire to improve is one of the major philosophies of alternative medicine.

Alternative medicine approaches patients as individuals whose total body health is related to the interaction between the body and mind. The main focus is on maintaining homeostasis, which is the body's natural tendency to maintain a biochemical and structural balance of hormones, enzymes, muscles, and organs to prevent disease or heal itself in times of stress. Alternative medicine focuses on the individual instead of his or her symptoms and seeks to optimize homeostasis by promoting healthy lifestyles, appropriate exercise, restful sleep, proper nutrition, and self responsibility.

There are numerous alternative medicine approaches; examples include acupuncture, applied kinesiology, Ayurvedic medicine, chiropractic medicine, aromatherapy, biofeedback, massotherapy, nutritional therapy, magnetic therapy, naturopathic and homeopathic medicine, reconstructive therapy, and traditional Chinese medicine. Numerous other fields exist in alternative medicine, and a good reference book is *Alternative Medicine, The Definitive Guide* compiled by the Burton Goldberg group. In the past few years, there has been much written about alternative medicine, and much public interest in exploring this medicine practice. Some recent studies have found that more and more people are choosing alternative medicine over conventional methods because of frustrations and lack of improvement with conventional treatments for pain.

Alternative medicine has been around for thousands of years, but with the establishment of the conventional philosophy of health in the past few hundred years, alternative medicine has constantly strived for credibility. There is much research and writing on alternative medicines, but because they are not considered equal to the scientific standards established by conventional medicine, alternative medicine is often inappropriately "accused" of lacking the science. Many doctors who specialize in alternative medicine require years of intensive training to become experts in their field, but many non-medical people have ventured into alternative medicine treatments with little or no experience, training or supervision which can contribute to the credibility problem.

My specialty, Physical Medicine and Rehabilitation (Physiatry) is actually a blend between conventional and alternative medicine strategies. My specialty uses a multi-disciplinary approach to a person, and I believe it is particularly suited for patients with chronic pain problems such as fibromyalgia. A knowledgeable physician who specializes in pain should use whatever works and not be limited to any particular treatment. Persons with fibromyalgia require individualized treatment programs, and creative strategies are necessary that blend together all types of treatments. I work together with other doctors and health professionals with the ultimate goal of helping patients achieve the lowest level of pain and highest level of function in spite of fibromyalgia.

This book is a detailed description of a philosophy and style of treatment for patients with fibromyalgia that blends various medicine components. This chapter is meant to highlight some specific alternative medicine approaches that I've used or am familiar with in the overall treatment of fibromyalgia.

Chiropractic Medicine

Chiropractic medicine is a type of alternative medicine proven to be very effective in treating back problems, headaches, and other pain disorders including fibromyalgia. Dr. Daniel David Palmer founded the modern chiropractic system a century ago in 1895, and today chiropractic medicine is the most popular field of alternative medicine. A key philosophy in chiropractic medicine is the holistic approach of the person with emphasis on the relationship between the spinal column, the nervous system, and the soft tissues of the body.

Proper alignment of the spinal column is necessary to achieve homeostasis and optimal health by allowing unimpeded nerve flow and neurologic and soft tissue function. If an imbalance, unequilibrium, or malalignment occurs in the vertebra or soft tissues, nerve pressure can occur. This results in altered signals which eventually lead to impaired nerve function and disease.

Chiropractic treatment can be effective in persons with fibromyalgia since patients have pain along the entire spinal functional unit which often responds to manual therapy. Manual therapy includes techniques that mobilize joints, improve range of motion, relax muscles, reduce muscle pain, and restore balance. These manipulations and adjustments are common manual medicine techniques performed by chiropractic physicians.

Manipulations are forceful movements of body parts to bring about a greater range of movement and to relax muscles. Adjustments are the application of a sudden and precise force to a persistent point in the vertebra or muscle to properly align the tissue. The desired outcome of properly aligned vertebra and muscles is improved balance, better neurologic flow, better circulation, and ultimately decreased pain and tension.

Many chiropractors use a device called an Activator to perform adjustments. This hand-held device has a spring loaded plunger mechanism which delivers focused pressure energy to a specific body part to achieve proper alignment. Chiropractic medicine also deals with the preventive, nutritional, strengthening, and fitness measures in helping individuals achieve their highest state of well-being.

I work closely with many chiropractic physicians in my community in the comprehensive treatment of patients with fibromyalgia. I believe the professional relationship and communication between chiropractic and medical physicians will continue to improve, and patients will benefit from the combined treatment approaches.

Acupuncture

Acupuncture originated in China thousands of years ago and has been successful in pain relief, particularly as an alternative to conventional pain relieving medication (analgesics). Acupuncture is based on the theory that energy pathways called meridians are present in the body that link the nervous system with the organ systems. There are multiple acupuncture points within these meridian systems that can be stimulated to improve the energy flow. These points can be stimulated using special needles, electrical stimulation, or pressure.

Acupuncture has been shown to stimulate the body's own natural pain killers, endorphins. It also affects neurotransmitters or hormones that transmit nerve impulses in a way that decreases the perception of pain. There are many studies that have shown the effectiveness of acupuncture as a substitute for surgical anesthesia.

There is a growing number of health professionals who have been trained in acupuncture and are practicing this technique in treating pain disorders. Many patients with fibromyalgia have benefited from acupuncture treatments. It is considered a potentially effective adjunct to a multi-disciplinary treatment approach.

Applied Kinesiology

Applied kinesiology focuses on the muscle activities with relationship to a specific problem. Specific muscles may be overactive causing a spasm, or underactive, causing weakness. When combined, these muscles can create a muscle dysfunction or imbalance causing pain and impairment. An applied kinesiologist uses procedures that strengthen weak muscles and relax tense muscles to help return injured or dysfunctional muscles to their normal state. It is felt that specific muscles are related to specific organs, and thus improving the muscle balance also improves organ function. Since patients with fibromyalgia have imbalances in their muscles due to portions of the muscles being overly tense and other portions being weak, applied kinesiology techniques can help many patients with fibromyalgia. Many chiropractors have learned applied kinesiology skills.

Magnetic Therapy

Magnetic therapy involves using magnetics to decrease pain by improving energy and blood flow in the body. Therapeutic magnets work on the same principle as acupuncture, but without the needle. Magnetic fields surround us, generated by natural mechanisms such as the earth, weather changes, or can be man made, such as the field seen in power lines and electrical devices. These magnetic fields can affect the body's function in both positive and negative ways by influencing the body's metabolism and oxygen availability to cells.

Magnets have two poles, a positive pole and a negative pole. It is felt that the positive pole causes negative effects such as decreased metabolic function and oxygen especially with prolonged exposure. The negative pole is felt to cause beneficial effects by normalizing the body's metabolic and energy functioning. Magnetic therapy can be used in numerous ways from magnetic strips applied to parts of the body to magnetic beds, pillows, and shoe inserts. Magnetic devices are very popular in Japan and Germany and are becoming increasingly popular in other parts of the world including the United States.

Some people believe that reduced exposure to the earth's natural geomagnetic fields can lead to a magnetic field deficiency syndrome which causes pain, headaches, insomnia, stiffness, and fatigue (sound like fibromyalgia?). People who spend a lot of time in buildings and cars are at risk of developing magnetic field deficiency syndrome. It is felt that magnetic therapy can be used to correct this deficiency and restore health.

Magnetic fields are used in diagnostic testing procedures such as MRI (magnetic resonance imaging), magnetic encephalography and nerve conduction studies to measure a body's structures and electrical activity safely and accurately. Magnetic field diagnostic techniques are already established in mainstream medicine, and therapeutic magnetic therapy is rising in popularity. It is considered a safe treatment, and many qualified health professionals are using magnets in their clinical practices.

Biofeedback

Biofeedback is a specific technique in pain management where individuals learn to control their body responses to achieve relaxation and pain relief. Unconscious bodily functions such as heart rate, pulse, digestion, blood pressure, brain waves, and muscle activity can be consciously controlled by increasing one's awareness of their autonomic nervous system function.

Seeking to decrease pain, an individual with fibromyalgia would train with a biofeedback device under the direction of a qualified biofeedback counselor. Biofeedback devices work by monitoring skin temperature, heart rate, muscle tension, electrical conductivity of the skin, or brain wave activity. These various devices measure body responses to stress and reflect the autonomic nerve activity. These devices also give a signal, (a noise, beep, or a visual reading) that the individual can monitor. The patient is then instructed on various techniques designed to achieve relaxation and observe for the body's desired responses as indicated by the biofeedback devices. The patient can be trained to accomplish the desired response. The more this learned response is practiced, the better the biofeedback skills become.

Biofeedback has the potential to be very effective in fibromyalgia, particularly in reducing stress, controlling headaches, and relieving muscle pain. It is also important as part of relaxation treatment for fibromyalgia (see chapter on Mentally Managing Fibromyalgia under the RElax and REfresh section). Biofeedback is essentially training a person to control his or her vital body functions using electronic devices that gives a person "feedback." This technique, when successfully learned, can be a powerful adjunct in controlling the pain and some of the problems associated with fibromyalgia.

Reconstructive Therapy

Doctors specializing in reconstructive therapy will determine what areas of the body are weak and damaged and might benefit from this form of treatment. A reconstructive solution, which usually contains a local anesthetic and a natural irritant such as phenol, dextrose, or other natural substance, is injected into the weak areas of soft tissues. This solution stimulates the healing response, particularly the formation of collagen, the major repair protein in the soft tissue region. This stimulated collagen growth can repair the weak and injured area and can increase strength, stability, and ultimately healing and decreasing pain. A wide range of musculoskeletal problems have been successfully treated with reconstructive therapy, usually at a fraction of the cost that would be required for medications, surgeries, and other therapies.

Massotherapy

Therapeutic massage has been used for thousands of years to treat various musculoskeletal problems causing pain and muscle spasms. Therapeutic massage, in addition to decreasing pain and spasms, helps decrease swelling, range of motion, and blood circulation. This type of alternative medicine has been a wonderful form of treatment in patients with fibromyalgia. Massotherapy is further described in the chapter on Physically Managing Fibromyalgia.

Nutritional Therapy

There has been a lot of recent research on the nutritional and biochemical aspects of fibromyalgia. This exciting area has the potential to be the new frontier cure in fibromyalgia research.

Conventional medicine has recognized the importance of diet in diseases such as diabetes, heart disease, gout, and osteoporosis. There has been more and more acceptance by conventional doctors on the important role that diet and nutrition plays in a person's overall health. Nutritional strategies can indeed play an important role in the overall treatment of fibromyalgia.

It used to be safe to tell individuals, regardless of their medical problems, to "eat well." This means eating well-balanced, nutritional meals which was thought to give a person adequate nutrients. However, eating the right foods does not necessarily ensure proper nutrition for a variety of reasons.

1) There are various toxins that contaminate our foods and may cause health problems.

2) The soil in which our food is grown has become deficient in minerals and vitamin nutrients over the years.

3) The refining process in preparing food causes loss of vital nutrients.

4) The American dietary pattern of eating refined fast-foods instead of natural fresh foods has resulted in deficiencies of certain vitamins and minerals.

There has been an explosion of nutritional products available on the market. The over-the-counter supplements and health foods are not subjected to the strict Food and Drug Administration (FDA) regulations as are prescription medicines. There have been instances where the FDA has warned consumers about contaminated health food products that cause medical complications, but, fortunately, these instances have been few. The FDA recently warned consumers about using dietary supplements that contain both ephedrine and caffeine, as this combination may cause serious adverse reactions such as heart attacks or hepatitis.

In understanding nutritional strategies, one must not assume that everything swallowed gets absorbed. The concept of bio-availability is important in health food products. *Bio-availability* is the ability of a particular product to be absorbed and used by a body.

Many factors are important in the bio-availability of a product: whether the particles can be dissolved and absorbed, whether the particles are small enough to pass through the cell membrane, whether the body digests these particles before they get absorbed, whether or not they are stable in the body, or whether the particles need to be attached to other particles in order to get absorbed.

Because of differences in bio-availability, the same product made by different companies can vary greatly in their ability to be absorbed and used by the body. In fact, very little of some products are actually absorbed by the body, making them ineffective, even though a particular company may advertise that its product is less costly.

What nutritional medicines are available in the treatment of fibromyalgia? Numerous studies have looked at biochemical abnormalities, oxygen abnormalities, hormone deficiencies, and other problems in trying to understand the pathogenesis of fibromyalgia. There have been various studies on nutritional replacements in fibromyalgia, and recent studies looking at magnesium and malic acid supplements have shown improvement in the patient's pain.

We do not know exactly how or why nutritional strategies may work in fibromyalgia. Some key ingredients in the body's biochemistry may be deficient, and they cannot perform various body reactions. Another theory is that the ingredients are present in sufficient quantities in the body, but are relatively deficient in areas that they are needed, or are used inefficiently in biochemical systems even if present. If less efficient biochemical pathways are used, this can result in more energy consumption, increased fatigue, and the production of byproducts that are considered toxic or painful. This combination of deficiencies and inefficiencies may lead to altered homeostasis and cause adverse reactions that ultimately produce fibromyalgia. I believe there are some basic principles in trying to optimize nutrition in fibromyalgia.

1) Eat at least three meals a day. This helps maintain proper energy for daily needs and keeps the body machinery working more efficiently. Those who are particularly bothered by irritable bowel syndrome may do better by eating six smaller meals per day to decrease nausea and abdominal pain.

2) Emphasize a diet that is low in fat, low in refined sugars, and high in natural fruits and vegetables.

3) Avoid caffeine, nicotine, and alcohol as these all interfere with the body's ability to manufacture energy and proteins and carry out efficient biochemical reactions.

4) Consider nutritional supplementation strategies. There are various alternative nutritional medicine strategies that include nutritional supplements, herbal medicine, juice therapy, enzyme therapy, and detoxification.

I encourage patients to be open-minded about their nutritional approach and to responsibly experiment. By this I mean that, before trying anything, be certain that it is a product made by a reputable company with good supporting data and references, and there is no risk of serious side effects. An average consumer needs to ask his or her doctor, nutritionist, pharmacist, and knowledgeable colleague, and read various articles to increase knowledge and be able to make decisions regarding various products. I don't recommend trying anything unless you know exactly what it contains, and your doctor assures you that these ingredients are not potentially harmful to your body.

Don't choose products because they have the best marketing strategies; base your decisions on your knowledge.

If a particular product is tried, then carefully monitor muscle pain, muscle stiffness, and body energy to see if there is any improvement. If you are undergoing numerous treatments for your fibromyalgia, it may be hard to tell if a nutritional approach is working, or if it is a combination of everything. Most of my patients, however, are able to report that nutritional strategies, if they are working, help by allowing them to reach a stable baseline with decreased frequency of flare-ups.

My philosophy is that you are allowed to try anything once. If you are not noticing any difference after a reasonable trial (for example, one month), this particular product probably will not work for you, and I don't recommend continuing with the same product. If some benefit is noticed such as decreased pain, improved energy, decreased stiffness, or overall feeling better, then the product should be tried another month and re-evaluated. You do not have to take any nutritional products for three to six months or longer before you notice any benefit; one month should be a long enough trial.

Find out from fibromyalgia colleagues what they have tried and what has worked for them. At our support group, whenever we ask what particular product has worked, we invariably get as many answers as there are people in attendance!

You need to find your nutritional balance. I do not think there are any magical nutritional approaches. Rather, there are effective nutritional approaches that can be part of overall successful treatment for fibromyalgia. Successful treatment of fibromyalgia involves a successful lifestyle change and improvement of well-being. Nutritional strategies are an important part of accomplishing this overall goal.

I have reviewed various types of alternative medicine strategies. There is no conventional or alternative strategy, or a blend of the two that cures fibromyalgia. As we doctors and patients continue to be open-minded and learn more about fibromyalgia and the cause and treatment, I anticipate more of a blending of conventional and alternative medicine strategies. A multi-disciplinary team approach works best, and I view the knowledge of a fibromyalgia doctor as the director of the "fibromyalgia production." You, the person with fibromyalgia, are the lead actor and are surrounded by a supporting cast, and the director. Instruction, guidance, and practice are allowed, but it is you that has to play and live the part. By taking an active role in your "fibromyalgia production," you will become part of your treatment solution, and not part of the ongoing problem.

Managing Flare-Ups

7

Every individual with fibromyalgia will experience flare-ups from time to time. Sometimes we can identify a specific precipitating factor, but many times we can find no reason for the flare-up. Flare-ups may be spontaneous or idiopathic meaning nothing specifically caused it; it just happened. One of the most frustrating complaints of fibromyalgia patients is that flare-ups occur in spite of doing everything right. Sometimes subtle factors can be identified that may be causing the flare-up, but many times there is no obvious reason for a flare-up. The patient must simply deal with them as they occur and try to accept that periodic, uncontrolled intrusions are part of this condition.

What exactly is a flare-up? How does one know if it is a flare-up due to fibromyalgia or if it is a new problem? What should we do during a flare-up; should we exercise, do our regular work duties, attend social events? These are frequent questions asked by individuals suffering from fibromyalgia. This chapter is a detailed guide to assist you in successfully overcoming a fibromyalgia flare-up.

My definition of a fibromyalgia flare-up is as follows: Increased regional or generalized pain or fatigue, when compared to a stable baseline level, that persists for at least 3 consecutive days and interferes with usual daily activities.

People with fibromyalgia experience increased pain on a daily basis. Fluctuations above and below our baseline state are typical - some days we feel better, other days we feel worse, and our pain moves around to different locations. Certain activities may cause a person to hurt more for a few days, but if the pain resolves or decreases to baseline, we would not consider this a flare-up.

Our tender points always have some degree of spontaneous soreness responsible for that "constant ache." Palpation of these tender points will cause increased pain, or certain activities will increase the pain, but the pain should quickly return to baseline. Flare-ups occur when the tender points become more persistently and painfully sore whether it be from known or idiopathic reasons.

If the increased pain persists for at least 3 consecutive days above the baseline level, then we need to begin specifically addressing our flare-up and asking various questions:

1. **Describe the pain.**
   Where is the pain? Is it localized to a region or is the whole body affected?
   When does it hurt? Is the pain constant or intermittent? If the pain is intermittent does it occur regularly in the morning, during the day, after exercise or at night? Intermittent pain can still meet the definition of a flare-up if it is "persistently intermittent" and interferes with daily functions.

2. **What caused this increased pain?** Many factors can cause flare-up including physical, emotional, environmental and idiopathic reasons. Not all pain is related to fibromyalgia, as other unrelated conditions can be present. If the pain is mostly in the morning, the factors may be related to poor sleep or poor sleep positioning. Increased pain during the day may reflect work activities, household activities, improper body mechanics. Pain after exercise may indicate that the person is overdoing or doing new and unusual activities or not adequately stretching and warming up before the exercise. Increased pain at night might reflect accumulated strains during the day from job activity, or may reflect strenuous leisure activity. Increased fatigue at night often causes increased pain. A person in constant pain may have a combination of multiple factors involved.

3. **What type of treatments can the individual do on his or her own?** If the cause or causes can be identified, they should be removed, altered or modified. Various stretches and exercises, resting certain body parts, restricting certain activities, are all a part of the personal strategies in dealing with a flare-up. Increasing the use of home modalities (heat, ice, etc.) or over-the-counter medications may help.

4. **When should your doctor be consulted?** Whenever a person has increased pain, whatever the reason, he or she can consult with the doctor at any time. People who have had fibromyalgia for a while learn that flare-ups are part of the condition and the doctor may not need to be consulted immediately,

but a home program can first be tried. However, even experienced fibromyalgia sufferers will get "new" pains or new problems that require further medical evaluations, so one is never discouraged from consulting with his or her doctor for any reason. If a person first tries to manage the flare-up on his own, the flare-up will either improve and return to baseline level, not improve, or change very little. If a flare-up does not improve, you will need to follow-up with your doctor (M.D., D.O., D.C.).

Your doctor will approach your increased symptoms with a basic question: Is this a fibromyalgia flare-up, or is a new condition involved? Your doctor will perform a clinical evaluation and determine if any specific diagnostic tests are needed. Part of the doctor-directed treatment might include prescription medicines, trigger point injections, therapy orders, manipulations, adjustments and specific instructions. Hopefully the program instituted will be successful in resolving the flare-up and enabling the person to resume his or her baseline fibromyalgia program.

I have just described a general basic format on how a fibromyalgia flare-up might be approached. The following sections of this chapter are descriptions and strategies using this general format:

1. **Where is the pain/flare-up? (body part)**
2. **Conditions that can cause the pain may be related or possibly related to fibromyalgia, or may be unrelated to fibromyalgia**
3. **Causes of this particular flare-up**
4. **Treatments to do on your own to resolve flare-up**
5. **Doctor strategies to resolve flare-up**

Each section represents a different part of the body with a highlighted diagram at the beginning for quick reference.

Headache

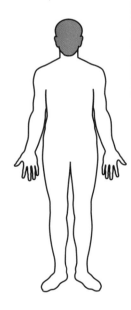

Conditions related or possibly related to fibromyalgia

- Tension/migraine headaches (the majority of fibromyalgia patients have these)
- Temporomandibular joint (TMJ) dysfunction (causes jaw pain, dizziness, and "head" pains; a common associated condition in fibromyalgia)
- Postconcussive syndrome (residual headaches, neck pain, difficulty concentrating after a concussion, often part of post-traumatic fibromyalgia and severe whiplash injury)
- Allergy flare-up with congestion or cold symptoms (allergies more common in people with fibromyalgia)
- Referred pain from tender/trigger points in neck and shoulder area
- Side effects from medications used to treat fibromyalgia (examples: tricyclic antidepressants, beta-blockers, migraine medicines, muscle relaxers)
- Hormonal changes in women (women with fibromyalgia commonly experience headaches as part of premenstrual syndrome [PMS] or menopause)
- Dry eyes syndrome (common in fibromyalgia; may cause eye irritation and headaches)
- Eye strain (eye muscles with fibromyalgia pain and fatigue cause headaches)

Conditions unrelated to fibromyalgia (but may cause headaches)

- Hypertension
- Renal disorder
- Infection
- Eye disease
- Cervical osteoarthritis (may cause secondary fibromyalgia, though)
- Vasculitis (inflammation of blood vessels)
- Cerebral hemorrhage
- Brain tumor
- Birth control pills

Isolate Cause(s)

1. Tension/migraine headaches
   a. Increased stress (personal relationship difficulties, job pressure, financial concerns, etc.)
   b. Exposure to bright lights, loud noises
   c. Dietary factors; certain foods such as cheese, chocolate, lunch meat, beans, alcohol, caffeine, and milk can trigger migraines. Cold foods ("ice cream" headache)
   d. Strenuous exercise-induced headaches
   e. Exposure to strong odors, chemicals, perfumes, fumes

2. TMJ dysfunction
   a. Grinding teeth at night (called bruxism)
   b. Chewing gum, hard candy, hard foods
   c. Jaw strain from excessive talking
   d. Yawning injury or "big bite" injury

3. Post-concussive syndrome
   a. Head injury from fall or car accident
   b. More sensitive to migraine headaches (see above)
   c. Usually co-existing neck muscle injury and pain

4. Allergy flare-up
   a. Exposure to pollens, molds, dust, etc.
   b. Sinus congestion or infection
   c. Sensitive to fumes, smells, viruses

5. Referred pain from neck and shoulder
   a. Strenuous physical activity (new job duties, move to new house, etc.)
   b. Weather related problems (cold, damp weather, shoveling snow, falling on ice)
   c. Spontaneous flare-up of tender/trigger points

6. Medication side effects
   a. Many medicines can cause headaches as side effects; new medicine or change in dosage
   b. Some medicines cause rebound headaches if they are stopped suddenly
   c. Fibromyalgia persons more sensitive to any medicine usually

7. Hormonal changes (probably altered "balance" of hormones, especially estrogen)
   a. Water retention phase of menstrual cycle causes exaggerated PMS (premenstrual syndrome) headaches in women with fibromyalgia.
   b. Menopause
   c. Estrogen medicines

8. Dry eyes syndrome
   a. Dry, dirty environment
   b. Contact lenses
   c. Sunlight sensitivity
   d. Chemical fumes sensitivity
   e. Cigarette smoke overexposure

9. Eye strain
   a. Prolonged reading
   b. Incorrect eyeglass strength
   c. Poor, artificial lighting

Treatments to do on Your Own

• Practice deep breathing and relaxation techniques; seek positive outcomes and strategies in dealing with stress or stressful relationships.

• Dampen and remove noises, use natural lighting especially in settings where a lot of reading and studying is required.

- Proper dietary habits, avoid skipping meals or prolonged fasting. Eliminate foods that you are sensitive to; be careful with food additives, caffeine and alcohol.

- Use over-the-counter medications such as aspirin, acetaminophen, ibuprofen, naproxyn; use medicines not only to treat pain but as a preventive measure (for example, take over-the-counter medicine one hour before exercise or a bothersome activity; women can take ibuprofen or a diuretic during the painful phase of menstrual cycle).

- Perform stretching and light conditioning exercises, avoid strenuous, heavy strengthening-type exercises. Place particular emphasis on stretching the neck and trapezius muscles.

- If dry eyes are the problem, avoid wearing contact lenses, use natural tears frequently, especially in smoky areas or dry environments. Review medications which may be causing dry eyes as a side effect. Stop smoking!

- Eye check-up. Determine if change needed in eye glasses; change reading habits to avoid prolonged reading time at once, especially if eye strain is a factor in causing headaches.

- Moist heat or ice to the back of the head and neck area

- Self-massage to work out soreness in the scalp muscle, jaw muscles and neck muscles.

If the flare-up does not return to baseline with these measures, see your doctor.

Doctor Strategies

- The doctor will discuss causes of headaches and the physical examination will focus on the nerves and soft tissues in the head and neck. The neurologic exam makes sure the reflexes, sensations, strength, eye muscles, visual acuity, face sensation, pupil reaction, hearing, swallowing, memory and orientation are all within normal limits. The palpation of the head and neck muscles to determine tender areas and testing neck and jaw range of motions to look for stiffness are also important components of the exam.

- Your doctor may order additional diagnostic testing which could include a head CT scan, EEG, head MRI, neuropsychological testing, X-rays of the sinus, TMJ, neck areas, and an eye examination. If the doctor feels that the headaches are due to flare-up of fibromyalgia or fibromyalgia-related factors, specific treatments directed at the headache can be instituted.

- If TMJ dysfunction is suspected, a referral to an appropriate dental specialist may be considered. TMJ treatment may include customized bite splints, crown and bridges as part of a restorative procedure, especially if there is a malocclusion.

- If eye-related headaches are a problem, a referral to an eye doctor may be needed. The eye doctor will evaluate vision and determine if glasses or adjustments are necessary. Vision therapy for strengthening the eye muscles can be helpful if headaches are induced by reading or eye strain.

- If allergies are involved, your doctor may prescribe a decongestant and an antibiotic. You may need to see an allergy specialist for specific testing or allergy shots.

- A variety of medicines may be used in treating headaches. These medications include analgesics, anti-inflammatories, muscles relaxants, anti-anxiety medicines, anti-depressants, such as tricyclics and serotonin reuptake inhibitors. Anti-migraine medicines such as Midrin, ergotamine tartrate, and an injectable medicine called sumatriptan can be very effective in treating migraine headaches.

- Trigger point injections might be tried especially if trigger regions are identified as the cause of the headache. The posterior occipital and cervical regions are frequently flared up and causing headaches, and may respond very well to a trigger point injection trial.

- Therapy modalities may be prescribed and might include hot packs, ultrasound, massage, craniosacral techniques, electric stimulation. Chiropractic treatment is helpful and includes manual therapy and adjustments.

- Biofeedback can help patients learn the relaxation response and control body responses that lead to headaches. Individuals can usually learn this technique after a few sessions.

- Hopefully these doctor measures will reduce the pain to a more stable and functional baseline, so you will be able to continue with your own home program.

Neck Pain

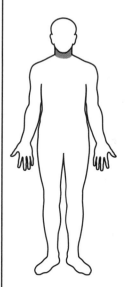

Neck pain often overlaps with headaches. Many people describe their headaches as in the back of their neck, radiating up to the base of their skull. However there is often a flare-up in the neck area, not necessarily associated with headaches.

Conditions related to or possibly related to fibromyalgia

- Cervical strain and sprain
- Flare-up of tender and trigger points in neck
- Referred pain from shoulder strain

Conditions unrelated to fibromyalgia

- Cervical disk disease such as degeneration or herniation
- Torticollis (wry neck or twisting of the neck due to abnormal muscles)
- Cervical osteoarthritis (may cause secondary fibromyalgia, though)

Isolate Cause(s)

1. Cervical strain and sprain
   a. Trauma such as an automobile accident where whiplash injury occurs; work injury, sports injury etc.
   b. Physical activities such as prolonged reading, driving, studying, looking up, or looking sideways; Examples: riding a bike with Ram's horn style handlebars; looking up; talking on phone hand-free by holding the phone with your head against your shoulder; turning head sideways

2. Flare-up of tender and trigger points in neck
   a. Weather changes, particularly cold, damp weather
   b. Increased stress, both physical and emotional
   c. Spontaneous, idiopathic

3. Referred pain from shoulder strain
   a. Repetitive reaching, overhead use of arms
   b. Lifting, shoveling, throwing, etc.

Treatments to do on Your Own

- Identify any physical causes and try to remove or modify these activities. If you notice certain head positions at work, such as turning your head to the right to look at a computer monitor or tilting your head to the side to hold up a phone so you can continue typing, you need to recognize that this is an aggravating position. Make the necessary changes such as rearranging work stations so that monitor is directly in front of you, get head phones if your job involves answering phones.

- Practice proper posture and fibronomics. Alternate various positions so as not to strain the neck muscles. Try to be consciously aware of the proper neutral position of the neck at all times (see Chapter 2 on Fibronomics).

- Continue a regular exercise program but emphasize neck stretching and range of motion. Do these exercises as warm-ups before starting a daily job or household chore.

- Take over-the-counter medicines including acetaminophen, ibuprofen, and naproxyn. Use muscle creams that give either heat or cold sensation. Use topical anesthetics such as capsaicin ointment.

- Use heat packs or ice packs, self-massage. Self-massage can make the muscles "hurt good." A soft cervical collar worn for short periods of time such as when driving or reading may help relieve the neck muscle pain.

If the flare-up does not return to baseline with these measures, see your doctor.

Doctor Strategies

- Your doctor will examine you with emphasis on the neck muscles, neck range of motion, and neurologic exam. If there is concern for underlying disk or arthritic disease, additional diagnostic tests may be ordered which include cervical spine X-rays, cervical CAT scan, MRI, or electro diagnostic testing.

- Specific treatments directed for fibromyalgia-related increased neck pain may include prescription medicine such as analgesics, anti-inflammatories, muscle relaxants. Trigger point injections using local anesthetic and cortisone combination may also be necessary, particularly if painful tender and trigger points are the major sources of the pain.

- Work restrictions may be needed to avoid repetitive neck movements from side to side or looking up or down. Your doctor will instruct you on proper neck posture.

- Specific therapies may include hot pack, ultrasound, massage, adjustments, cervical collar, and neck exercises. Traction can sometimes help, but many people with fibromyalgia find that cervical traction increases their neck pain. (A therapy course may average 3 times a week for a month as needed.) Chiropractic treatments may help.

- Hopefully these doctor measures will reduce the pain to a more stable and functional baseline, so you will be able to continue with your own home program.

Shoulder Pain

Conditions related to or possibly related to fibromyalgia

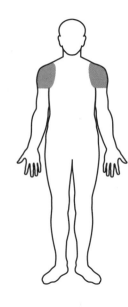

- Shoulder strain, rotator cuff tendinitis (tendinitis common in fibromyalgia patients)
- Biceps tendinitis (inflammation of tendon in upper arm flexion muscle)
- Shoulder bursitis (inflammation of bursa or fluid-filled sac in shoulder)
- Shoulder adhesive capsulitis (inflammation and tightening of the shoulder joint lining – also called frozen shoulder)
- Reflex sympathetic dystrophy (condition where the small sympathetic nerves to the arm become overstimulated)
- Flare-up of tender and trigger points in shoulder area

Conditions unrelated to fibromyalgia

- Rotator cuff tear
- Neurologic referred pain from radiculopathy (inflamed nerve root), brachial plexus injury, (shoulder nerve group) or shoulder nerve entrapment
- Shoulder dislocation
- Shoulder arthritis

Isolate Cause(s)

1. Shoulder strain
   a. Physical activities that involve a lot of reaching or use of the arms in outstretched or overhead position. Example: cleaning windows
   b. Activities requiring throwing or lifting such as bowling, softball, weight-lifting, shoveling snow
   c. Seat belt trauma following an accident
   d. Shoulder pressure from a heavy backpack or narrow bra strap
   e. Driving a car with a stick shift; prolonged driving

2. Rotator cuff tendinitis, biceps tendinitis, shoulder bursitis
   a. Throwing, weightlifting, shooting activities
   b. Repetitive reaching or pushing on the job
   c. Yard work requiring clipping and trimming
   d. Putting up holiday decorations
   e. Fall on outstretched arms (rotator cuff injury)

3. Shoulder adhesive capsulitis (frozen shoulder)
   a. Shoulder injury which leads to decreased use of shoulder and stiffness
   b. Shoulder inflammation (tendinitis, bursitis)

4. Reflex sympathetic dystrophy
   a. Shoulder injury
   b. Shoulder inflammation
   c. Nerve irritation (radiculopathy, carpal tunnel syndrome, autonomic nerve hypersensitivity)

5. Flare-up of tender and trigger points in shoulder area
   a. Excessive physical activities - example: carrying heavy suitcase
   b. Stress
   c. Weather changes (cold, damp); weather-related activities (shoveling snow, holiday decorations)

Treatments to Do on Your Own

- Remove or modify physical activities that are causing shoulder pain. Reevaluate your work station or house duties to minimize shoulder reaching, lifting or overhead use.

- Follow proper fibronomics; remember to keep the arms close to your body when performing tasks involving reaching or overhead use of the arms.

- Perform regular shoulder stretching and flexibility-type exercises. Examples:

   1. Reach your arms overhead as far as possible and hold for three seconds.
   2. Perform shoulder rolls for 15 seconds each side several times a day to loosen the shoulder soft tissues.
   3. Do corner stretches. Stand in a corner and put each hand on the wall at shoulder level and do a reverse push-up into the corner, feeling the muscles between the shoulders stretch and "hurt good."

- Wear a strapless bra or a bra with wider straps to minimize focused strain and pressure on the trapezius muscles.

- Use moist heat, try an ice pack, use muscle creams and self-massages frequently to shoulder muscles.

- Continue a regular exercise program but emphasize neck stretching and range of motion. Do these exercises as warm-ups before starting a daily job or household chore.

- Take over-the-counter medicines both to treat the pain and as a preventive measure. Take the medicine one hour before you will be performing activities that may aggravate your shoulder; that way the medicine will be absorbed and start to work right when you need it.

- Avoid using a sling as this increases the tendency for stiffness and weakness in the shoulder and makes the rehabilitation process more difficult.

If the flare-up does not return to baseline with these measures, see your doctor.

Doctor Strategies

- Your doctor will focus on the shoulder exam which will include shoulder palpation, checking range of motion, and evaluating shoulder stability. He will check whether or not there is any impingement or tear of the rotator cuff. The shoulder muscles will be examined to look for muscle spasms, painful tender points or swelling. In addition the neurologic exam (reflexes, sensation, and strength) will be evaluated to look for any underlying nerve damage.

- Depending on the exam results the doctor may order additional diagnostic testing including shoulder X-ray, shoulder arthrogram, shoulder MRI, and electro diagnostic testing.

- If the increased shoulder pain is thought to be related to fibromyalgia, specific treatment including medications (analgesics, anti-inflammatories, and muscle relaxants) can be tried.

- Trigger point injections and shoulder injections can be helpful. Injections into muscle, joint space, tendon or bursa can help, depending on the location of the pain. "Spray and stretch" is a good technique for shoulder pain, in which a vapo-coolant is sprayed onto the skin followed by stretching and manipulative therapy. Chiropractic treatments such as manual therapy and adjustments are also helpful.

- Therapies emphasizing the shoulder area can include hot pack, ultra-sound, electric stimulation, iontophoresis, massage, shoulder stretching, strengthening, and mobility exercises.

- Work restrictions may be necessary which would include avoiding and minimizing repetitive reaching and overhead work, decreased lifting with the arms, and decreased operation of hand controls.

- Hopefully these doctor measures will effectively control the flare-up and reduce the pain to a level which can be managed on your own.

Elbow and Arm Pain

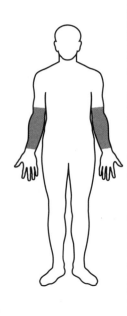

The dominant side will usually flare up more compared to the non-dominant side.

Conditions related to or possibly related to fibromyalgia
- Lateral epicondylitis (tennis elbow)
- Medial epicondylitis (golfer's elbow)
- Elbow strain
- Forearm strain
- Flare-up of tender and trigger points

Conditions unrelated to fibromyalgia
- Cervical radiculopathy (inflamed nerve root in neck)
- Brachial plexopathy (irritated shoulder nerve group)
- Carpal tunnel syndrome (pinched nerve in wrist)
- Ulnar nerve entrapment (pinched nerve in elbow)
- Fractures

Isolate Cause(s)

1. Lateral epicondylitis (tennis elbow)
   a. Playing tennis
   b. Repetitive power gripping i.e. hand tools
   c. New job activities requiring more forearm stress such as squeezing objects or bending the wrist back.

2. Medial epicondylitis (golfer's elbow)
   a. Sometimes from playing golf!
   b. Power gripping with the wrist bent in (wrist flexion).

3. Strains/flare-up of tender and trigger points
   a. Any new or unusual physical activity involving the arm (job, hobby); examples: writing numerous letters or bills; ironing for a few hours.

Treatments to Do on Your Own

- Remove or modify activities that cause or aggravate the symptoms.
- Use the unaffected arm to make up for some of the function the painful arm usually does.

- Continue a regular exercise program but emphasize stretching the elbow and forearm, especially before any activity.
- Use over-the-counter medications for increased pain as a preventive measure.
- Continue a regular exercise program, (emphasize arm stretching and range of motion).
- Do these exercises as warm-ups before starting a daily job or household chore.
- Put the arm in very warm water and soak and stretch.
- Do self-massage techniques with pressure and rubbing of the tender regions of the elbow and forearm; use muscle creams and get either a hot or cool effect along with the massage.
- Follow fibronomics and proper body mechanics.

If the flare-up does not return to baseline with these measures, see your doctor.

Doctor Strategies

- Your doctor will examine you and pay particular attention to the elbow and forearm area. The palpation exam will cover the epicondyle area (tennis elbow and golfer's elbow regions), as well as palpation of the forearm muscles. Range of motion will be checked in the elbow and wrist joints to determine if there is any inflammation. The neurologic exam (reflexes, sensation, strength, and coordination) will also be tested to make sure there is no underlying neurologic disorder or nerve entrapment.

- Certain tests may be considered including X-rays and electrodiagnostic testing. If inflammation is present and thought to represent an underlying inflammatory disease, laboratory studies may be ordered.

- If the flare-up is thought to be from fibromyalgia, specific doctor treatments may include instruction on ways to rest and exercise the affected area. There may be job restrictions that limit the use of the affected arm or arms or specifically limit the amount a person may lift, grasp or operate hand controls. Your doctor will reinforce the need to use the unaffected side to compensate for the affected side until the pain quiets down, but also to be careful not to overuse the good side so as not to cause pain there also.

- Medication to be considered include anti-inflammatories, pain medicines, and muscle relaxants. Injections may also be appropriate, particularly into painful or trigger areas.

- Specific therapies may include ultrasound, with cortisone, electrical stimulation, friction massage, elbow braces (such as a tennis elbow brace) and specific stretching and strengthening exercises. Chiropractic adjustments may also be effective.

- Hopefully these doctor measures will effectively control the flare-up and reduce the pain to a level which can be managed on your own.

Wrist and Hand Pain

Conditions related to or possibly related to fibromyalgia

- Writer's cramp
- Wrist strain
- Wrist and hand tendinitis
- Autonomic nerve hypersensitivity (small sensory nerves are easily "irritated" especially in hand and cause pain, burning, swelling, itching, etc.)
- Reflex sympathetic dystrophy (condition where the small sympathetic nerves to the arm become overstimulated)
- Flare-up of tender and trigger points in the wrist and hand

Conditions unrelated to fibromyalgia

- Carpal tunnel syndrome (pinched nerve in wrist)
- Peripheral neuropathy (disease of the small nerves causing numbness, weakness and loss of reflexes)

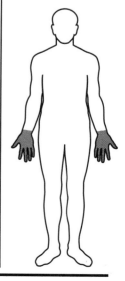

- Cervical radiculopathy (inflamed nerve root in neck)
- Fracture
- Rupture of tendon
- Arthritic conditions
- Dupuytren's contracture (tightening and scarring of the connective tissue in the palm)
- Upper motor neuron disease (disease of the brain or spinal cord)

Isolate Cause(s)

1. Repetitive job activity, particularly those that require a lot of gripping or grasping, operating tools, and repetitive wrist movement
2. Increased writing, typing, or computer-keyboard operation
3. Exposure to cold temperature; changes in temperature
4. Spontaneous flare-up from areas that refer pain to the wrist and hand

Treatments to Do on Your Own

- Remove or modify the activities that cause the pain.
- If unable to remove or modify the activities, alternate between various tasks or use the more unaffected arm as often as possible without causing any increased pain on that side.
- Do specific exercises for the wrist and hand. Maintain proper body mechanics and fibronomics.
- If cold temperature aggravates the symptoms, wear gloves when working outdoors or in cool, wet environments.
- Use over-the-counter medicines to treat pain or as a preventive measure, taken 1 hour before the "offending" activity.
- Continue a regular exercise program but emphasize neck stretching and range of motion. Do these exercises as warm-ups before starting a daily job or household chore.
- Use muscle creams if they do not cause increased sensitivity.
- Use hot or cool water or alternate between the two to create your own contrast bath. Prepare a bowl of hotter water and a bowl of ice water. Dip painful hand into bowls, alternating one minute of heat with 30 seconds of cold for a total of 10 minutes; do this twice a day.
- If the flare-up does not return to baseline with these measures, see your doctor.

Doctor Strategies

- Your doctor will perform an examination that will emphasize your wrist and hand areas. The exam will consist of examining the joints to see if there is any evidence of inflammation such as swelling or limitation of motion. There will be an examination to see if there are trigger points where the fingers lock in a bent position. The neurologic exam will be important to make sure there is no evidence of carpal tunnel syndrome or radiculopathy, or other nerve problem that can cause hand pain.

- Further testing may include laboratory studies, X-rays, electrodiagnostic testing, or a bone scan.

- Specific treatments related to fibromyalgia may include medications such as analgesics, anti-inflammatories, or muscle relaxants.

- Injection of the wrist or carpal tunnel area with cortisone may help. Bracing of the wrist in the neutral position can be helpful particularly if wrist strain or tendinitis is a major problem.

- Various therapies that can be tried include modalities such as heat, electric stimulation, massage, stretching, exercise programs, more bracing. Chiropractic adjustments of the wrist have been effective.

- Epidural blocks or sympathetic blockade are two anesthesiology techniques that may be appropriate, particularly if there is extreme autonomic (small nerve pain) hypersensitivity. Shoulder-hand syndrome or reflex sympathetic dystrophy can occur in fibromyalgia. This condition is characterized by overactive autonomic and small sensory nerves that cause extreme pain, burning and swelling in the hand especially.

- Hopefully these doctor measures will effectively control the flare-up and reduce the pain to a level which can be managed on your own.

Chest Pains

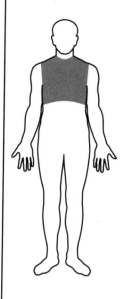

Conditions related to or possibly related to fibromyalgia

- Costochondritis (rib pain)
- Pectoralis (chest muscle) strain
- Mitral valve prolapse (bulging of one of the heart valves)
- Anxiety/panic attacks
- Referred symptoms from irritable bowel syndrome
- Fibrocystic breast disease
- Flare-up of tender and trigger points
- Sensitivity to environmental allergens/asthma

Conditions unrelated to fibromyalgia

- Coronary artery disease
- Hiatal hernia
- Esophagitis (inflammation of the esophagus)
- Pneumonia
- Bronchitis
- Asthma
- Peptic ulcer disease

Isolate Cause(s)

1. Coughing-induced flare-up of chest wall muscle
2. Smoking
3. Increased physical activities involving a lot of reaching, twisting, or pulling; example: washing the car
4. Breast pain from pregnancy, large breasts, or breast implants
5. Lactating breasts, causing increased strain/irritation of breast tissue/muscles
6. Anything that provokes anxiety attacks such as stress, sensitivities to certain foods or beverages, exercise, chemicals
7. Anything that aggravates allergies, such as ragweed, pollen, chemicals, fumes, and dust

Treatments to Do on Your Own

- Identify, remove and modify any causes, for example if a new job activity requires a lot of reaching forward with the arms outstretched, modify the work area so that excessive reaching and subsequent chest irritation does not occur.
- Add stretching exercises that focus on the chest wall and pectoral muscles.
- Practice deep breathing exercises and relaxation techniques.
- Chest pain is usually very disturbing to patients especially if it is a new symptom. Although there are many ways it can be attributed to fibromyalgia, many people feel that there is a problem with the heart and will consequently see their doctor immediately. If you are having new onset of chest pain, always see your doctor at once. If you have previously had chest pain attributed to your fibromyalgia and you have a flare-up, you may try these techniques first. If your pain is not returning to baseline with the measures you try on your own, see your doctor.

Doctor Strategies

- Your doctor will focus on your chest exam which includes listening to the lungs and the heart, checking blood pressure, pulse, respirations, and palpating the chest muscle areas. Additional specialist referral may need to be considered (cardiologist, pulmonologist, gastroenterologist or obstetrician).

- Testing that could be considered includes laboratory studies, chest X-ray, EKG, cardiac echogram, cardiac stress test, cardiac angiogram, pulmonary function test, bone scan, thoracic spine X-rays, mammogram, allergy testing.

- If the chest pain is thought to be related to the fibromyalgia, specific treatments may include allergy shots (if allergies are a problem), medications, including analgesics, anti-inflammatories, muscle relaxants, anti-anxiety and anti-depressant medicines. These treatments may help decrease the offending conditions (allergies, anxiety, muscle spasm etc.) that cause chest/breathing difficulties.

- The patient will often have soreness in the chest wall area, particularly the designated tender point of the second rib, and an explanation that this is not the heart may help decrease some of the anxiety associated with these chest symptoms.

- Injections can be helpful into the costochondral regions using a combination of local anesthetic and cortisone. Chiropractic adjustments have been effective. Therapy to include modalities and chest wall exercises can help. Stretching and strengthening exercises using large rubber bands (Therabands) have been particularly effective for decreasing chest wall pain by increasing chest muscle flexibility and strength. If anxiety attacks are a particular problem, referrals for biofeedback and stress management may be considered in addition to the other treatments.

- Hopefully all of these measures will help return the pain to a stable baseline that can be managed on your own.

Back Pain

Conditions related to or possibly related to fibromyalgia

- Strain of back or hip muscles
- Scoliosis (frequently seen in fibromyalgia patients)
- Irritable bowel syndrome (which can cause referred pain to the low back and sides)
- Flare-up of tender point and trigger point in the back

Conditions unrelated to fibromyalgia

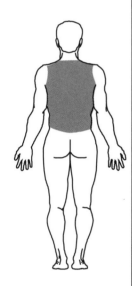

- Osteoarthritis/osteoporosis (may cause secondary fibromyalgia, though)
- Degenerative disk disease
- Herniated disk
- Spinal stenosis (narrowing of the spinal canal)
- Spondylolisthesis (forward displacement of one vertebrae upon another)
- Compression fracture
- Subluxation syndrome (imbalance of vertebral, soft tissue and nerve positions)
- Bone tumor
- Scarring from previous back surgery
- Connective tissue disease
- Foot/leg problems causing bad alignment

Isolate Cause(s)

1. Strain
   a. A new or unusual physical activity that requires bending, twisting or lifting, whether at work or at home
   b. Prolonged walking or standing especially on hard surfaces
   c. A recent long car ride without any rest stops, especially if driving
   d. Playing an unusual sporting activity, such as a basketball game or volleyball
   e. Sleeping in a different bed on a surface that was either too hard or too soft; sleeping on stomach
   f. A specific trauma from heavy lifting or improper body mechanics
   g. Coughing or sneezing spells
   h. Poor fitting shoes or high heels

2. Spontaneous flare-up of tender and trigger points
   a. Weather changes, especially cold, damp weather
   b. Recent flu or a viral infection
   c. Increased emotional stress

Treatments to Do on Your Own

- Remove or modify the offending physical activities, if possible.
- Evaluate the work station and make changes to reduce back strain.
- Pay attention to proper body mechanics and fibronomics.
- Alternate between various positions such as walking, standing or sitting and avoid being in one position for too long. Sit whenever possible at work.
- Review your exercise program and continue exercises that emphasize back stretching.
- Use modalities, particularly a hot tub or moist heat to the painful back muscles; sometimes ice works well. Use these modalities as frequently as needed.
- Have a spouse or significant other rub muscle cream into the back or do a massage.
- Do your own back massage by rubbing your back against a door knob or a golf ball on the floor, or devices to provide deep trigger point pressure.
- Take over-the-counter medicine as a preventive and therapeutic measure; that is, take it one hour before an "offending" activity to try to prevent pain, or take it when you have more pain.
- Continue a regular exercise program but emphasize neck stretching and range of motion. Do these exercises as warm-ups before starting a daily job or household chore.
- Temporarily wear a back brace, and if work particularly aggravates back pain, consider using a back support for work only.
- Consider a cushioned insert in the shoes to absorb some of the ground reactive forces and prevent them from aggravating the back. Orthotics or special foot braces may help.
- Stand on a rubberized mat at work to reduce some of the force from the hard surface.
- Try to eliminate excessive body weight, particularly in the abdominal area as abdominal obesity is a major cause of increased strain on the lumbar muscles.
- Make sure you are sleeping on a comfortable bed that supports your back, paying attention to proper sleeping position to enable the back to rest at night.
- Extra rest during the day for acute back flare-up.
- If the flare-up does not return to baseline with these measures, see your doctor.

Doctor Strategies

- Back pain is one of the most common symptoms a doctor evaluates. Your doctor will examine you particularly to rule out some serious causes of back pain such as a herniated disk or radiculopathy. The exam will include palpation of the spine and spinal muscles and measuring the back's flexibility and range of motion. The neurologic exam performed will assess reflexes, sensations, muscle strength and coordination to look for nerve damage. Straight leg raising is a technique that can sometimes help to determine if there is acute nerve root irritation.

- Depending on the exam findings, additional testing may be necessary. Some testing may include laboratory studies, back X-rays, back CAT scan, lumbosacral MRI, electrodiagnostic testing, bone scan, myelogram.

- If the condition is thought to be related to fibromyalgia, specific treatment will likely include instruction on proper rest, exercise, and activity. Work restrictions may be necessary such as restricting the amount of weight able to be lifted, or restricting bending and twisting, or requiring alternating between various positions. Lighter duty work may be necessary on a temporary basis. Depending on the severity of the flare-up, time off work for recovery and therapy may be recommended.

- Various medications including analgesics, non-steroidals and muscle relaxants may be considered. Trigger point injections, spray and stretch techniques, and lumbar epidurals are additional ways of providing pain relief.

- A therapy program may be prescribed to include:
    a. Modalities such as hot packs, ultrasound, electric stimulation and ice
    b. Massage and massotherapy
    c. Back stretching and conditioning exercises, and
    d. Instruction on a home program

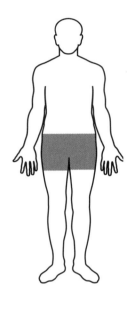

- Chiropractic manual adjustments may also be helpful. Often a combination of all of the above works best.
- Hopefully these doctor measures will reduce the pain to return to a more stable and functional baseline so you will be able to continue with your home program.

Hip/Pelvis Pain

Conditions related to or possibly related to fibromyalgia

- Sacroiliac strain
- Gluteal strain (buttock muscle)
- Lumbosacral pelvic dysfunction (back-pelvic muscle imbalance)
- Tension myalgia of the pelvic floor (tight pelvic muscles)
- Greater trochanteric bursitis (hip bursa irritation)
- Ischial tuberosity bursitis (buttock bursa irritation)
- Coccygodynia (tailbone pain)
- Spontaneous tender and trigger point flare-up in hip/pelvic area
- Irritable bowel syndrome (refers pain to pelvic area)
- Endometriosis (refers pain to pelvic area)
- Irritable bladder (can cause pelvic pain)

Conditions unrelated to fibromyalgia

- Hip osteoarthritis
- Avascular necrosis (deterioration of the hip joint due to lack of blood supply)
- Piriformis syndrome [compression of sciatic nerve from piriformis (muscle in the lower buttock)]
- Sacroiliitis (inflammation of the sacroiliac joint)
- Radiculopathy, plexopathy or other nerve irritation in lumbosacral area
- Abdominal and pelvic diseases
- Hernia

Isolate Cause(s)

1. Excessive bending or twisting due to various physical activities that may be occurring on the job or at home. Example: carrying boxes up and down steps
2. Prolonged walking and standing, especially on concrete surfaces or uneven surfaces
3. Hamstring tightness which alters the lumbosacral pelvic balance and rhythm
4. Prolonged sitting, especially on a low seat
5. Excessive climbing, especially stairs
6. Standing on ladders for long periods of time
7. Sleeping on stomach or poor sleep positions

Treatments to Do on Your Own

- Identify offending activities and try to remove or modify them.
- Emphasize back and pelvic stretching exercises, work on the hamstrings to get them as stretched out as possible, as the more flexible they are, the better the lumbosacral pelvic joints can be balanced.
- Use heat, such as hot packs, hot baths, hot tubs, or try ice.
- An aquatics exercise program in a heated pool, emphasizing stretching and walking for preventive and therapeutic treatment.
- Continue a regular exercise program but emphasize neck stretching and range of motion. Do these exercises as warm-ups before starting a daily job or household chore.
- Over-the-counter medicines
- Cushioned shoe inserts
- Tight, wide belts to stabilize the sacroiliac joints (leather weight-lifting belt can work well)
- If coccygodynia or tailbone pain is a problem, try sitting on a ring or donut cushion and take it wherever you go for your chairs and car seat.
- If endometriosis pain is a problem particularly during the water retention phase of menstrual cycle, try taking an over-the-counter diuretic along with ibuprofen.
- If these measures are not helping your flare-up return to baseline level, see your doctor.

Doctor strategies

- Your doctor will examine you with emphasis on the low back, hip and pelvic areas. Particular attention will be paid to the sacroiliac area to see if it is in proper alignment, or if it is out of balance and demonstrates increased pain when various sacroiliac stressing maneuvers are performed. Palpation of the back and hip bones and muscles to see if there is particular increased tenderness, as well as palpation of the gluteus maximus (buttock muscle) tender points and other muscles is emphasized. Referral to an obstetrician or gastroenterologist may be necessary for pelvic or abdominal problems. Sometimes a hernia can be present which can require referral to a surgeon. If a urologic disorder is suspected, a referral to a urologist may be recommended.

- Additional testing can include pelvic and hip X-rays, bone scans, pelvic CAT scan, electrodiagnostic testing, pelvic ultrasound, and abdominal studies.

- If the pain is directly related to fibromyalgia, specific treatment programs may include:

    a. Medications (anti-inflammatories, non-steroidals, muscle relaxants)
    b. Trigger point injections and specific sacroiliac injection
    c. A therapy program including ultrasound, hot packs, electric stimulation, iontophoresis
    d. A sacroiliac corset and manual adjustments may help stabilize the low back and pelvis and help realign the sacroiliac joint.
    e. Lumbosacral pelvic stretching and strengthening exercises are often useful to help tight muscles to relax and strengthen weaker muscles to stabilize the lumbosacral rhythm.
    f. Aquatic exercises are particularly effective.

Hopefully, these doctor measures will help reduce the flare-up to a more stable baseline that you can manage on your own.

Knee/Leg Pain

Conditions related to or possibly related to fibromyalgia

- Knee strains, bursitis or tendinitis
- Tender or trigger point flare-up in knees or legs
- Restless leg syndrome (leg pain and restlessness especially at night)
- Referred pain from myofascial regions and back, hip and sacroiliac regions

Conditions unrelated to fibromyalgia
- Deep venous thrombosis (blood clot in leg)
- Peripheral vascular disease (blood vessel hardening or blockage)
- Neurologic irritation in leg
- Chondromalacia patella (knee cap pain from arthritis or degeneration)
- Osteoarthritis
- Knee ligament, cartilage, or meniscus injury
- Bone fracture

Isolate Cause(s)

1. Increased hill climbing, walking, standing, kneeling or crawling.
2. Increased running activities as can occur when one begins a jogging, walking, or bicycling program, or uses a stair machine.
3. Increased squatting; example: playing volleyball at a picnic causes thigh pain.

Treatments to Do on Your Own

- Avoid or modify activities that are aggravating the condition; reduce the amount of time spent on your feet.
- Avoid running activities, decrease your running and walking program in half until baseline level is achieved. Then gradually increase the program again, but not to the point where you had been before so as not to cause another flare-up.
- Wear a neoprene knee brace when more active on feet.

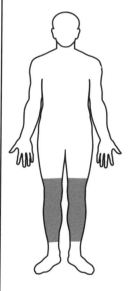

- Review the exercise program and focus exercises on stretching the knees and calf muscles.
- Foot orthotics, good supportive but comfortable shoes for work and exercise.
- Use over-the-counter medicines for preventive and therapeutic pain control.
- Continue a regular exercise program but emphasize leg stretching and range of motion. Do these exercises as warm-ups before starting a daily job or household chore.
- Rubbing legs at night, moving legs around especially if restless leg syndrome is a problem.
- Modalities such as hot packs or whirlpool, or ice the knees especially after activity.

If these measures are not helping your pain return to baseline level, see your doctor.

Doctor Strategies

- The knee exam involves palpating for any tender areas, swelling, or heat. The knee joint itself is examined for any evidence of instability that might indicate an internal derangement or ligament strain. Testing the knee motion and searching for any unusual clicking or grinding is performed. Your doctor will make sure there is no swelling in the calf or veins, and check for adequate pulses and nerve function.

- Depending on your doctor's concerns, additional testing may include venus duplex scan to look for a blood clot, vascular studies to measure for arterial disease, knee and leg X-rays, or knee arthroscopy, especially if internal knee derangement or tear is suspected.

- If the condition is related to fibromyalgia, specific doctor treatments may include direction on proper exercises. Certain restrictions such as avoiding bending at the knees, kneeling, repetitive stair climbing, may be necessary. A therapy program that includes knee strengthening exercises may be instituted. Knee braces can be ordered, and knee injections and various medicines, especially anti-inflammatories and analgesics, may be tried. For restless leg syndrome, drugs such as Klonopin or Sinemet may be tried.

Hopefully these doctor measures will help decrease the pain to a stable baseline that you can manage again on your own.

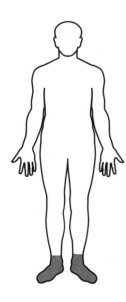

Ankle/Foot Pain

Conditions related to or possibly related to fibromyalgia
- Ankle sprains and tendinitis
- Foot tendinitis
- Plantar fasciitis (bottom of foot)
- Autonomic nerve hypersensitivity in feet (causes pain, burning numbness)
- Spontaneous flare-up of tender or trigger points
- Referred pain from painful back, hip, leg areas

Conditions unrelated to fibromyalgia

- Referred pain from radiculopathy or other nerve lesions
- Tarsal tunnel syndrome (pinched nerve at the ankle)
- Peripheral neuropathy (disease of the smaller nerves causing numbness, weakness, loss of reflexes)
- Morton's neuroma (a painful nerve "scar" between the toes)
- Plantar warts
- Athlete's foot
- Stress fracture
- Arthritis, bunions, spurs
- Connective tissue disease
- Vascular disease

Isolate Cause(s)

1. Walking for long periods of time, and walking on hard surfaces, such as concrete or uneven surfaces; example: mall shopping for hours
2. Running activities (jogging, sprinting)
3. Prolonged standing (shopping, waiting in line, job)
4. Jumping activities (volleyball, basketball)
5. Trauma to the feet (dropping something on the foot or twisting foot on stone)
6. New shoes or poorly fitting shoes

Treatments to Do on Your Own

• Modify or remove aggravating activities. Get off feet as much as possible.
• Wear cushioned inserts, heel pads or metatarsal pads.
• Try home modalities, such as heat, alternately dipping the feet between warm and cold water, foot whirlpool.
• Continue a regular exercise program but emphasize neck stretching and range of motion. Do these exercises as warm-ups before starting a daily job or household chore.
• Rest, specifically get off your feet and elevate them.
• Wear comfortable shoes that have been broken in.
• If these measures do not reduce the pain to baseline, see your doctor.

Doctor Strategies

•Examination of the ankle and feet will include checking pulses and skin to look for any vascular disease. Palpation of the ankle and foot tendons to look for specific areas of soreness, making sure that the joints move to their full range, and making sure that the sensations, strength and reflexes are all normal, are key components of the examination. Specific testing might include X-rays and bone scan. A podiatry referral may help.

• Various treatments include:
    a) instruction on exercises and rest
    b) medications
    c) orthotics, whether they be soft cushioned ones or more firm supportive ones
    d) therapies including ultrasound, electric stimulation, or iontophoresis may be helpful.

Hopefully these doctor measures will reduce the pain to a baseline that you can manage on your own.

Whole Body Flare-Up

Patients will more often complain of the whole body flaring up rather than one specific region. The overall pain can be overwhelming, but usually the person can isolate specific areas that are worse than others. The combination of increased pain and fatigue can be particularly difficult for people to cope with and try to maintain their daily functional activities.

Various conditions related to fibromyalgia or possibly related to fibromyalgia can be responsible for a whole body flare-up. Usually a combination of conditions exist. Categories of these conditions include:

a. Ideopathic or spontaneous flare-up of tender and trigger points
b. Tendinitis and bursitis
c. Trauma (strains, sprains)
d. Aggravation of hypersensitive autonomic nervous system by various stress factors
e. Localized or regional flare-up that became generalized

Isolate Cause(s)

1. Increased emotional stress [new job, job promotion (with additional responsibilities), job transfer, job termination, new house, divorce, newborn, death in family, illness in family]

2. Increase or decrease in physical activities; new job duty, "weekend athlete," "weekend yard warrior," decreased usual exercise program, illness

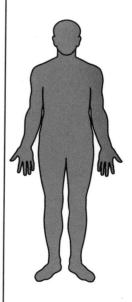

3. Weather changes: In my practice I see flare-ups occurring most commonly in the Fall, then Winter, then Spring, and least often in Summer. There may be no other cause except for cold, damp weather. The Fall is a particular problem because warm days end with cold, damp evenings. These extremes of temperature fluctuations cause problems in fibromyalgia because the weather change actually "stresses" the muscles and small nerves (autonomic nerves) and causes a flare-up. Another major Fall fibromyalgia enemy is the Holidays with its associated physical and emotional stresses that make us particularly prone to flare-ups (see Managing Flare-ups).

4. Trauma. This can be a localized strain which ultimately causes a generalized flare-up, or it can be an unrelated trauma such as a fracture, which heals, but that region becomes more painful and contributes to a generalized flare-up.

5. Surgery. Surgery for any reason can cause flare-up. This is probably due to various factors including stress, strains related to all the required positioning that is unusual for the body, and possibly from general anesthesia. A temporary bedridden state and a relative deconditioning can occur due to inactivity caused by surgery.

   Carpal tunnel surgery, knee surgery, hip surgery are common procedures that often flare up fibromyalgia. Any surgery and surgery related restrictions on activities or weight-bearing will disrupt the "baseline" body mechanics and put patients at risk for a generalized fibromyalgia flare-up. I have seen patients with generalized flare-ups occurring after silicone breast implant surgery and rupture of the implants, presumably due to an inflammatory reaction against the silicone.

6. Infection. (Flu, cold, bronchitis, etc.) Getting a flu shot has caused flare-ups in many patients of mine.

7. A flare-up of allergies especially in people who have multiple environmental allergies; allergy flare-ups can occur with exposure to dusts, pollens, weeds, chemicals, fumes, sprays, etc. Flare up risks increase during allergy seasons such as Spring and Fall.

8. In women, flare-ups can be associated with hormonal changes related to the menstrual cycle or menopause.

9. Depression: Depression is common in fibromyalgia and can contribute to a generalized persistent flare-up.

10. Seizures: I have several patients with seizure disorders and fibromyalgia who experience flare-ups after having a generalized seizure. The resulting muscle spasms during the actual seizure causes increased muscle strain and pain.

11. Pregnancy (see The Fibromyalgia New Mother)

Treatments to Do on Your Own

I think it is important to try to isolate your worst area or areas and focus on them according to the guidelines described for different areas.

- If you are anticipating a situation that could cause a flare-up such as an upcoming surgery or pregnancy, try to prepare yourself for this "event" by paying extra attention to stretching and light conditioning exercises to get your muscles in as good shape as possible (see Chapter 3 on Physically Managing Fibromyalgia). Ask your doctor what to expect physically: position required during surgery; how long; post-surgery limitations, etc. so you can best prepare yourself and avoid "surprises."

- However, if you are reading this now, chances are you are already experiencing a flare-up and don't have much use for preventive measure at this point. You can try to remember the preventive measures the next time!

- Identify emotional stresses and practice relaxation techniques and stress reduction strategies.

- Make a list of all your daily physical activities and look at each one individually to try to determine whether there has been any recent change in this type of activity that may be a factor in causing or contributing to your pain. If you can identify specific activities, try to remove or modify them temporarily. More importantly, make permanent adaptive changes in these activities.

- In menstruating women who have problems during the water retention phase, take a diuretic and anti-inflammatory medicine for pain such as ibuprofen during your worst week of the menstrual cycle.

- Take over-the-counter medicines regularly until your flare-up is under control, then try to minimize your need for medications.

- Soak in a hot tub or take hot baths or frequent long, hot showers, self-massage your most sore muscles.

- Massotherapy for extra work on the muscle spasms and pain.

- Try soft tissue and muscle nutritional supplements, particularly those that contain supplementary doses of magnesium, malic acid, manganese, vitamin B1 and vitamin B6.

- Continue your routine exercise program at a reduced level if necessary. It is very important to continue with your stretching and conditioning exercises no matter how bad you feel. It is okay to reduce the intensity of your usual programs, say for example you decrease by one-half the time and number of repetitions. Not doing anything will cause the muscles to suddenly experience a deconditioned state which contributes to even more muscle pain in addition to your current flare-up.

- If these measures and strategies indicated in the other sections for specific areas are not helping you return to your baseline, see your doctor.

Doctor Strategies

- Your doctor will want to make certain that you are not experiencing pain due to another problem. Various diseases can aggravate preexisting fibromyalgia, and fibromyalgia can be secondary to an underlying connective tissue disease, thyroid problem, inflammatory arthritis, or other problem. Attention will be paid on the exam to various tender points and whether or not there is any evidence of inflammation, spasm, or neurologic problem. If there is concern about an underlying medical problem other than the fibromyalgia, various testing, including laboratory and X-rays may be ordered. Further consultants may be involved, and if depression is a problem, there may be a referral to a psychiatrist or psychologist.

- Various doctor strategies for managing a flare-up include worker activity restrictions, instruction on exercises, medications, manual therapy, and other therapy programs that include modalities, myofascial release techniques, massage, exercises, and development of a successful home program. If specific areas are identified as more troublesome and more painful, these particular areas will probably receive extra attention. The goal is to try to get the pain reduced as quickly as possible, and then to reactivate the muscles to get them to their functional baseline and keep them there.

When the Pain Doesn't Settle Down

8

What do you do when the flare-up does not settle down to your baseline as you had hoped? You may have identified causes, taken steps on your own, followed up with your doctor and the treatments, and yet the pain has not abated. The flare-ups usually quiet down to baseline over time, but sometimes this does not happen.

There are various reasons why one's pain level will flare up and stay at a higher level. One reason is that there may be a new trauma superimposed on a previous stable fibromyalgia. This new trauma causes permanent escalation of the baseline level of pain and may involve new areas of pain not previously present. This trauma may be from an automobile accident or work injury. It may be more subtle from cumulative (wear and tear) trauma as can be seen with jobs that require repetitive activity. Over time, this cumulative micro trauma can lead to permanent increased pain.

Worsening can also be related to progressive arthritis (osteoarthritis or degenerative joint disease) that may aggravate fibromyalgia. There is a subset of individuals whose fibromyalgia may worsen in later years from degenerative joint disease, which can cause increased pain from altered mechanical forces, inflammatory reactions, or even biochemical changes. Tendon, ligaments, and bursa also undergo degenerative changes over time, and may cause associated fibromyalgia flare-ups and worsening.

Treatments may be partially effective but the previously remembered baseline is not achieved. He or she remembers what it was like to have lesser pain, and this "remembered standard" is what is expected of successful treatment. When this "remembered standard" is not achieved, the perception is that the treatment is failing and there may be increased anger, frustration, anxiety and depression.

It is often frustrating for the doctors as well since we want to help patients achieve the pain reduction that they wish. If this does not happen, we have to review the treatment approach and be faced with the probable realization that this may be the best it gets. Assuming that additional factors or problems unrelated to fibromyalgia have been ruled out, there often comes a time when a doctor may have to say "this may be the best it gets and I don't have any further treatments to offer at this time." This is very difficult to hear as patients always want something else to try. They may ask, "can I try this?" or "what else can I do?" and sometimes the difficult answer is "there is nothing further to do at this time."

Addressing the issue of a chronic and permanent problem is very difficult, and it needs to be handled with compassion and hope. I try to emphasize to the patients that their pain is not their fault or caused by something they are doing wrong. Even in patients who have not been compliant with the recommended treatment program, I do not confront them, but give them their options and respect the choices and decisions they wish to make regarding their fibromyalgia. In the end, the management of fibromyalgia is the responsibility of each individual and I try to teach self-responsibility which includes accepting the level of pain that is present and trying to get on with life as fully as possible.

Acceptance of the fibromyalgia is a most difficult issue as addressed in Chapter 4, Mentally Managing Fibromyalgia. It is hard enough to try to accept the fibromyalgia, but to try to accept a permanently higher level of pain or the realization that there are no magical treatment options available, may be too overwhelming for some individuals. Counseling may be recommended.

Even knowledgeable physicians have to say "I don't know" at times when asked what the future will hold for any individual and his or her pain.

I emphasize the importance of continuing with a regular program in spite of the pain. Probably the pain would be even worse if the regular modalities, stretching and exercises are not done. I also believe that individuals who are knowledgeable about their condition and follow through with a responsible home program will have a greater chance of controlling their pain and decreasing it over time. Also, we are learning more and more about fibromyalgia and its treatments, and new discoveries will ultimately create newer and more successful treatment strategies. These factors are good reasons to have hope.

Individual job situations need to be addressed. As a rehabilitation specialist I have always adhered to the philosophy that we should focus on our abilities and not on our inabilities. The word "rehabilitation" means to make able again, and I try to emphasize abilities in spite of fibromyalgia. Preserving the job or some modified version of it is a high priority since patients with fibromyalgia who are not working usually report just as much pain and see me just as frequently as patients who are working. It is important to accept the condition, make the adjustments, and follow through with a regular home program.

In spite of all of our best efforts, there will be times when people with fibromyalgia will be disabled by this condition. In surveys, individuals with fibromyalgia rank their condition as more disabling than individuals with rheumatoid arthritis, heart disease, lung disease, and other chronic disorders. Even though fibromyalgia is not a disease, it has potential to cause significantly debilitating effects on an individual's life, and there may be impossible situations that prevent a particular individual from working, thus rendering him or her disabled. The disability factor should be addressed only as a last resort and needs to be a decision that is mutually arrived at by both patient and doctor.

Long term follow-up studies on patients with fibromyalgia who have been rendered disabled or awarded a legal settlement have shown that the majority of them continue to be bothered by fibromyalgia and seek medical treatment for this condition. So there is no question that the debilitating effect of fibromyalgia persists even if jobs are stopped, stresses are relieved, or lifestyles are altered. However, the majority of people with fibromyalgia do not reach this severe disabling state and I believe we can further decrease the number of those who do reach this disabling end point by aggressively identifying and treating fibromyalgia as early as possible.

How I Approach the Fibromyalgia Patient

9

Since I began private practice in August of 1988, I have seen thousands of patients with fibromyalgia. As a physician specializing in physical medicine and rehabilitation (physiatrist), and as a patient who has fibromyalgia, I have a special interest in researching and treating this condition. Over the years the strategies I use to approach persons with fibromyalgia have evolved based on experiences and new information. This chapter will give you some insight into my clinical approach of the fibromyalgia patient. This information should assist you in choosing the physician who will treat your fibromyalgia.

I tend to initially approach fibromyalgia by a treatment strategy I call the "full court press." This strategy means attacking the fibromyalgia from different directions including education, medication, therapy, massage, trigger point injections, biofeedback and nutritional aspects. No one treatment works 100%, but each treatment can work to some degree and, when combined, the person can often notice a fairly substantial reduction in their pain level. Using the basketball analogy for full court press, multiple treatments are designed to apply "pressure" on the fibromyalgia and try to find an "opening" in the pain.

People with fibromyalgia have had this condition for a long time and they want to see quick initial success with any treatment. If only one treatment at a time is slowly and gradually introduced, the patient may become discouraged or feel that the small percentage of improvement is not substantial in his overall condition. This could lead to increased frustration, anxiety and impatience. I think it is better to use the full court press strategy because it is easier to back off certain treatments, especially if there is some initial improvement, than it is to gradually introduce one or two treatments at a time over a longer course. There is more psychological advantage to achieving the quickest, most successful response possible. I make sure I individualize the treatment approach so as to avoid overwhelming the patient. In other words, overwhelm the fibromyalgia, not the person!

There are four categories of fibromyalgia patients that I see in my private office setting. They are:

1. **The newly diagnosed fibromyalgia patient with no previous treatment.**

2. **The previously diagnosed fibromyalgia patient who is referred for additional recommendations or follow up of initial treatment approaches.**

3. **The fibromyalgia patient who is experiencing a flare-up.**

4. **The chronic fibromyalgia patient who has been resistant to multiple treatment approaches.**

Each fibromyalgia patient is a unique individual who has specific problems and needs. There is no generic patient, so to speak, but there are similar problems that occur and specific treatment strategies and goals that can be successful in most individuals. Whereas there may be limited patterns and strategies, there are unlimited individualized approaches that can be developed. I simply try to find whatever works best for a given individual.

I will describe some specific approaches for each category. It is not possible to include every specific or possible approach. The following is meant to be a general guideline on how I specifically approach fibromyalgia patients from my personal perspective as a physiatrist.

A physiatrist is a specialist who is trained in diagnosing and treating the patients with disorders causing functional limitations (for example, fibromyalgia). The primary treatment goal is to achieve the highest level of function and quality of life possible. The physiatrist has a unique perspective in that he or she takes a holistic approach to the patient and uses all available resources to obtain the best possible outcome. In someone with fibromyalgia, the physiatrist would try to help the individual have the least amount of pain and the greatest amount of function in spite of having a disorder that causes ongoing pain.

1. The new fibromyalgia patient with no previous treatments

First, a detailed history and physical examination is performed. I ask about characteristic complaints related to muscle pain, tender points and associated conditions. I listen for two "diagnostic" complaints: "I hurt all over" and "my pain moves around." The physical exam emphasizes the muscles and tender points. I use the tender point criteria as a guide, and the diagnosis of fibromyalgia is made based on the best diagnosis that fits the complete clinical picture.

Because there may be associated subclinical connective tissue or thyroid abnormalities, I will usually order laboratory studies that includes sedimentation rate, blood count, ANA, rheumatoid factor and thyroid studies. If any of these are abnormal, I will entertain a different diagnosis altogether with possible secondary or reactive fibromyalgia. If there is concern about a neurologic problem such as carpal tunnel syndrome or radiculopathy, I may order additional testing such as X-rays or electrodiagnostic testing.

An individualized treatment program is initiated which includes:

Education: Discussing what is fibromyalgia and my treatment philosophy, and letting the patient identify realistic goals and expectations. I provide written and video information on fibromyalgia. Each patient is told that fibromyalgia cannot be cured or eliminated, but it can be controlled with treatments. The expected realistic outcome in the treatment of fibromyalgia is not the complete elimination of pain, but rather the reduction of pain to a lower, more functional baseline, even though some pain will be chronically present.

Medications: I often prescribe sleep modifiers, especially if poor sleep is a problem. I may use anti-inflammatories and/or muscle relaxants depending on the presence of any "inflammation" and muscle spasms. I may also begin a tricyclic anti-depressant or a serotonin re-uptake inhibitor medicine. Soft tissue nutritional supplements can also be prescribed at this time. I instruct on potential benefits and side effects of each medication.

Therapy program: I usually recommend a therapy program to find what treatments will work and instruct the person on an individualized home program. I emphasize heat, stretching, myofascial release, massage, light conditioning, and proper body mechanics including fibronomics.

Work strategies: If the person works at a job or within the home, we review ways to minimize strain and trauma to the various muscles. This involves reviewing fibronomics, proper posture and body mechanics and any potential work restrictions and adaptations.

I will arrange a follow-up appointment, usually within a month, to review a person's response to the initial treatment. I instruct the patient on calling me prior to the visit if there are any questions. Many of my patients' therapy programs are performed under my direct supervision so I am able to monitor them and make any changes as needed.

2. Previously diagnosed fibromyalgia patient

If the patient is referred by another doctor for additional fibromyalgia recommendations, I take a detailed history and examination. Previous laboratory tests, X-rays and treatments are reviewed. If appropriate, I confirm the diagnosis of fibromyalgia.

If the patient is returning for follow-up evaluation to determine response to initial treatments, I would review their interim history and determine what treatments may be effective. If labs or studies were performed, these are also reviewed at this time. If a different condition is suspected, appropriate studies, referrals, and treatments are initiated, depending on the condition.

In the patient with confirmed or previously diagnosed fibromyalgia, I review what the patient's understanding of fibromyalgia is at that point, and what has worked so far. I try to identify strategies the patient has done on his or her own at home and at work, and whether these strategies helped.

Medications may be adjusted. If certain medicines were tried and not effective, different ones and different combinations can be tried. Anti-depressants will especially be considered if the patient is demonstrating a depressed mood. If depression is a serious problem, referral to a psychiatrist or psychologist may be done.

If a limited number of painful areas are causing the majority of pain, I would consider trigger point injections using a local anesthetic and/or cortisone for therapeutic purposes. Trigger point injections are often helpful in relieving pain in more flared-up areas and allowing other treatments to work more effectively, even long after the trigger point injection wears off.

It appears that part of the long-term effectiveness of trigger point injections relates to the ability to desensitize or disrupt the tender points. Even though the actual effects of the medicines used may wear off within hours, the improvement in the pain may persist for weeks.

Therapy approaches are determined by what has worked or has not worked so far, and I try different strategies with emphasis on soft tissue therapy, massage, and developing a successful home program of stretching and light conditioning. Manual therapy may be considered, I frequently refer patients to chiropractic physicians and we work together in helping the individual patient achieve the lowest level of pain or the lowest baseline possible. I frequently order biofeedback for relaxation and stress management. I feel massotherapy is very effective in treating fibromyalgia.

I encourage people to optimize their nutritional status and consider soft tissue nutritional supplements. I also discourage cigarette smoking as this increases pain in fibromyalgia.

I will arrange for a follow-up if I have begun a formal treatment program, so I may reassess the progress and make any further treatment changes as needed.

3. Fibromyalgia flare-ups

The fibromyalgia patient with flare-up is asked to identify the area or areas of flare-up, and whether it is a generalized flare-up. (See Chapter on Managing Flare-ups.)

A cause will be searched for, whether it arises from work, home, changes in the weather, changes in sleep patterns, personal stresses, or spontaneous (idiopathic).

A discussion on what has been tried already by the patient is important. The previous medicines and treatments will be reviewed. A detailed history is important when assessing a flare-up.

The physical examination will focus on identifying the cause or causes of the flare-up and make certain that no new problem unrelated to fibromyalgia is occurring. If an unrelated problem is suspected, further testing and treatment will follow as appropriate for this condition.

If fibromyalgia is indeed the culprit in the flare-up, an individualized treatment approach will focus on the following factors:

Education: Identifying a cause and trying to modify or avoid it.

Medications: Pain relievers, NSAID's, muscle relaxers, trigger point injections (especially if there are limited number of areas causing most of the pain).

Therapies: Emphasis on soft tissue work and more acute measures for the specific area of flare-up. If appropriate, a referral to an additional doctor, such as a chiropractic physician, for further specialized treatment as part of the entire rehabilitation program. A follow-up is scheduled to re-evaluate progress and make any additional recommendations. The main treatment goal for flare-ups is to resolve the flare-up and enable the individual to return to a stable baseline level of pain that can be successfully managed on his or her own.

4. Chronic fibromyalgia patients resistant to multiple treatments

Unfortunately there are patients who have had multiple appropriate treatments, but continue to be bothered by significant pain associated with fibromyalgia. The pain is disabling for them in the sense that they are not able to carry out their daily activities or job functions. Chapter 8 is specifically devoted to addressing the fibromyalgia patient who is resistant to treatment.

A history and physical examination are performed. Many times a person is injured or becomes unemployed and disabled because of the resistant fibromyalgia. But the converse is often true. That is, the unemployed and/or disabled individual will more likely have chronic fibromyalgia which is resistant to treatment.

Treatment considerations for the chronic resistant fibromyalgia patient include:

a. New medications or medicine combinations

b. Chronic pain management techniques involving a multi-disciplinary team approach; addition of a psychologist, physical therapist, nurse, doctor, occupational therapist, and dietician to the treatment team

c. A fibromyalgia support group referral

d. Referral to a different doctor for a different opinion or treatment approach

e. Address work or disability issues

f. Supportive counseling and reassurance

No matter what category the fibromyalgia patient may fit, I always try to find some way to improve the person's quality of life in spite of the pain. Some people have better results with treatments than others, but I believe everyone with fibromyalgia can find something that works no matter how bad they feel.

The Fibromyalgia Worker

10

Fibromyalgia plays an important role on the job. Whether the fibromyalgia was actually caused by work injuries, or whether the work is aggravating the pre-existing fibromyalgia, the worker has to make changes in the way he or she approaches work to minimize pain and functional impairment. Post-traumatic fibromyalgia due to work injuries is being seen more frequently. There may be a single trauma such as a back strain from lifting, or it may be a cumulative trauma that appears over time from continuous performance of specific job activities. The number of cumulative trauma cases has increased because of improved technology causing jobs to be more repetitive and performed with increased speed, more specialized work places, and more awareness of the symptoms by workers and physicians.

There are various risk factors involved in developing post-traumatic fibromyalgia or aggravating pre-existing fibromyalgia. These risk factors include:

1. **Repetitions:** Jobs that require a lot of repetition put continuous strain on soft tissues. Many manufacturing and assembly line jobs and secretarial jobs involve frequent use of the hands and arms and are examples of jobs that are risky due to the number of repetitions.

2. **Excessive force:** Jobs that require excessive force also increase the risk. Activities such as power gripping or movements against gravity (lifting objects off the ground or pushing up on tools) are examples of activities requiring excessive force on the muscles.

3. **Unnatural positions:** If joints are not in the neutral or natural position, more strain is exerted on these joints and soft tissues. The arms outstretched or overhead, elbows away from the body, wrists bent up or down, palms facing up, or leaning forward and bending are various unnatural positions that increase the risk of injury and subsequent post-traumatic fibromyalgia.

4. **Cold damp environments:** Jobs that require a lot of outdoor exposure, particularly in the winter time, changing temperatures within the job itself (going from a freezer to a refrigerator to a heated area at various times during the course of the day) will increase fibromyalgia symptoms.

5. **Stress:** Increased stress on the job can occur for a variety of reasons. Working long hours or overtime, working strictly night shift, worries about job security or financial issues, and extra responsibilities in management positions are a few examples of stresses on the job that increase the risk for fibromyalgia symptoms.

Various work categories exist and are determined by the amount of lifting and carrying required. They range from sedentary work to very heavy work (see table).

Often, light duty is still not tolerated well by individuals with fibromyalgia. Even though there is not heavy lifting involved, the work involves a lot of arm repetitions which can increase pain in people with fibromyalgia.

There are a lot of things an individual with fibromyalgia must consider when looking for a job. First, one must develop a realistic outlook for the type of job that he or she would qualify for from a physical standpoint. Since individuals with fibromyalgia have a difficult time performing activities that require reaching, overhead use of the arms, bending and heavy lifting, there are certain high risk jobs that would not be considered realistic. Examples of high risk jobs involving a lot of reaching and overhead use of the arms include assembly line jobs, dry-walling, hairstyling, secretarial, computer programming, transcription, carpentry and bricklaying. These types of jobs are more demanding on the neck, shoulders and upper back.

Examples of jobs that require a lot of bending and heavy lifting include construction workers, welders, truck drivers, and movers. These jobs are more demanding on the low back. You need to know the risk factors and risky jobs and try to avoid them as much as possible when looking for a job.

Work Categories

SEDENTARY WORK: Lifting 10 pounds maximum and occasionally lifting and carrying such articles as dockets, ledgers, and small tools. Jobs are sedentary if walking and standing are required only occasionally and other sedentary criteria are met.

LIGHT WORK: Lifting 20 pounds maximum with frequent lifting and/or carrying of objects weighing up to 10 pounds. Requires walking or standing to a significant degree, or sitting with a degree of pushing and pulling of arm and/or leg controls.

LIGHT MEDIUM WORK: Lifting 30 pounds maximum with frequent lifting and/or carrying of objects weighing up to 20 pounds.

MEDIUM WORK: Lifting 50 pounds maximum with frequent lifting and/or carrying of objects weighing up to 25 pounds.

MEDIUM HEAVY WORK: Lifting 75 pounds maximum with frequent lifting and/or carrying of objects weighing up to 40 pounds.

HEAVY WORK: Lifting 100 pounds maximum with frequent lifting and/or carrying of objects weighing up to 50 pounds.

VERY HEAVY WORK: Lifting over 100 pounds, carrying objects over 50 pounds frequently.

Work categories

Know your strengths and weaknesses, and know that, in spite of fibromyalgia, you can be a reliable, dependable, efficient and intelligent worker who would be an asset to any company. Research the companies and fields that particularly interest you and take advantage of any professional guidance that might be available through various schools and career centers. There are many reference books that will have necessary information. Let your natural ability to be organized, concise and perfect help you in developing a professional resume and plan.

Explore the type of hours available at any prospective job. Part-time, flexible hours might suit you best compared to a full-time job. Swing shifts and strictly night jobs are more difficult for patients with fibromyalgia due to the disruption it causes on the already impaired sleep pattern. Even persons who work permanent night shifts never develop the quality of sleep as compared to persons that work the day shift, so keep this in mind and seek stable daytime hours if you can.

Health insurance is certainly an important issue. Persons with fibromyalgia require periodic medical attention ranging from seeing the doctor, taking medication, participating in therapies, to taking time off work altogether. A job that provides adequate health insurance and acceptable sick time is certainly a plus.

A frequently asked question is whether an individual should reveal to a potential employer that the individual has fibromyalgia. I always advise my patients not to volunteer any information regarding their health, specifically as it relates to fibromyalgia, because chances are a potential employer will not know what fibromyalgia is and will consider it something negative. The Americans with Disability Act, otherwise known as ADA, protects people who have disabilities from job discrimination. A potential employer is not supposed to ask about any medical condition, either on the application or during the interview, according to the ADA.

I understand how both the potential employer and potential employee have specific interests and concerns. The employer does not want to hire someone who may have a pre-existing medical condition that will worsen once the individual begins a new job, thus costing the employer. From this standpoint, any medical information the employer can learn about the employee would probably be more helpful to the employer and more harmful to the employee, particularly if the employer were to assume that fibromyalgia, because it causes pain, would mean that the employee would not be able to perform a particular job. On the other hand, the potential employee wants to be honest and not hide anything, yet does not want to reveal anything that would cost him a job, particularly if the potential employee is perfectly capable of performing the job.

As an advocate for the patient, I feel the potential employee should receive the benefit of the doubt or have the more slightly favored position. By this, I mean the individual with fibromyalgia who is seeking a job should not reveal that he or she has fibromyalgia to a potential employer. By law, this question should never come up before a job is offered, but if it does, the individual needs to answer in the manner that he or she is most comfortable. If the individual chooses to reveal that he or she has fibromyalgia, it should be done in a manner that focuses on the abilities in spite of fibromyalgia, not the inabilities because of the fibromyalgia. If you reveal that you have fibromyalgia, I would try to convince the employer how you have a good understanding of your condition and know your limitations. Discuss how you feel you are capable of handling the job and that you consider yourself a responsible, reliable and efficient individual who would be an asset to the company. An honest and confident approach is probably your best long-term strategy even though this approach could still "scare off" some potential employers. But don't offer anything about your fibromyalgia unless you have to.

Once an individual finds a job, what can be done to prevent fibromyalgia from developing or flaring up? An approach to the fibromyalgia worker or worker at risk for developing post-traumatic fibromyalgia includes a program that emphasizes proper body mechanics, preventive measures, early treatment of injuries, and ongoing training and education.

Proper body mechanics involve following ergonomics and fibronomics. As we have learned, ergonomics is a scientific study of the relationship between the human body and work. It involves designing work task capabilities of the human body to minimize the risk of injury. To decrease the risk, one tries to reduce the number of repetitions by taking more frequent breaks, rotating jobs, working at a slower speed. Force can be reduced by modifying tools or using power tools, relocating switches, and using gravity to work with you and not against you.

Following proper body mechanics is the key. One tries for the neutral or natural position by keeping the arms at the sides and below the shoulders, avoiding twisting of the forearms and bending of wrists, adjusting tools and not wrists, adjusting the height of chairs or tables, and modifying the work station to keep everything within reach.

Protect your low back during lifting. Before lifting or moving any object, test the weight to make sure it can be moved safely. Use an assistive device or another individual whenever necessary, and if two or more individuals are involved, make sure that there is effective communication to reduce the chance of a sudden jerk or a dropped load.

Mentally plan every move prior to the actual lifting. Always use a wide balanced base of support, keeping the back in its normal arched position when lifting. Always remember to bend at the knees and hips and keep the load as close as possible to the body. The head and shoulders stay up as the lifting movements begin to help maintain the arch of the lower back and tighten the stomach muscles. Use the legs to do the lifting, standing up in a smooth, even motion to decrease the lower back stress.

Minimize twisting of the back. Whenever a direction change is necessary when carrying a load, always move the feet or pivot in the direction of change. This reduces the twisting at the waist and thus reduces the strain and stress on the back.

There are various techniques for lifting loads. The following diagrams demonstrate four examples: a modified diagonal lift, one knee lift, the golfer's lift, and straight leg lift.

Modified Diagonal Lift:

The modified diagonal lift is used for lifting heavy items which are one or two feet off the floor. Establish a wide stance with one foot in front of the other. Placing yourself slightly over the item, bend at the hips and at the knees. With the head and shoulders up, straighten the knees and hips to lift the object off the ground.

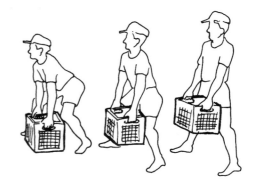

One Knee Lift:

Place one foot beside the front portion of the object to be lifted; drop slowly to other knee. Grip object firmly at near and far corners with head and shoulders up and lower back arched, then lift or roll the object onto top of thigh. Maintaining same posture, stand with object cradled. (This lift should be avoided by persons with knee problems.)

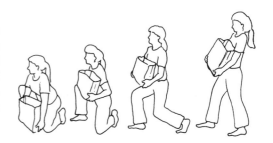

The Golfer's Lift:

Used by people with knee problems, decreased leg strength, or when they must lift where there is a barrier in front of the item (such as a railing or deep storage container). Place one hand on table or other fixed object to support upper body; arch the back, bend at hips and raise one leg behind; by raising one leg, the upper body weight is counterbalanced and forward bending of the low back is reduced. To pick up item, the individual should look up, push off with free hand, and lower raised leg.

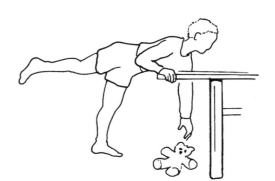

Straight Leg Lift:

This lift is used when knees and hips cannot be bent. Position body as close to the object as possible. If reaching over something into a lower work area, press legs forward against object over which you are reaching. While bending slowly at hips, (not the waist) you should firmly grasp item and bring it closer if necessary. With the low back arched and head up, the lift is completed by rotating hips backward into a full standing position.

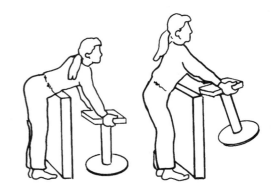

Preventive measures focus on stopping the problem from ever developing in the first place, or in the case of the fibromyalgia worker, preventing flare-ups from occurring. Maintain a regular stretching and exercise program to reduce the chance of injury. A worker should approach his or her job the same way a trained athlete approaches a sporting event. Prior to attempting any running or whatever activity the particular sport calls for, the athlete will perform warm-up exercises, especially those that include stretching. The fibromyalgia worker must also perform warm-up stretching exercises prior to performing the daily "event." The stretching exercises will improve flexibility and circulation, decrease the tendon tightness, and decrease the chance of stretch and tear injuries.

Examples of simple stretching and warm-up exercises are shown on the next page. This will include neck rotations, back bends, side bends, overhead reaches, wrist stretches, fist stretches, hand shake downs, and shoulder rolls. (see Chapter 3 - Physically Managing Fibromyalgia, for more examples of stretches.)

These exercises should be done before work, during break, and after work. Pay special attention to home activities, as outside or recreational activities can cause significant strain on the muscles. For example, doing home carpentry work, laundry, or bowling twice a week may be aggravating fibromyalgia more than the actual work activities. Try to neutralize the home activities.

If fibromyalgia symptoms begin to flare up, early attention to these symptoms is needed. The company doctor or nurse should be notified. Contact your personal physician, if available. Over-the-counter pain medications, modalities (heat, ice or muscle creams) and work restrictions can be part of the initial treatment. If the flare-up worsens or a new problem develops in spite of your approaches, further medical evaluation by your own physician will be necessary. The earlier that a flare-up or injury is treated, the better the chance of resolving the problem.

Ongoing training and education involves periodically analyzing your work site and recognizing and correcting any ergonomic or fibronomic hazards. Work positions, power tools, ergonomic chair, telephone headset, or other adaptive equipment may be helpful.

Working with your company's safety committee to review any injury trends or identify any patterns that can be further analyzed and remedied, if possible, is part of the ongoing follow-up needs.

The employee, the employer and the doctor can work together to devise strategies at the work place that invite cooperation. The Americans with Disabilities Act requires employers to provide equal employment opportunities for people who are able to do the job, but who are limited by physical disabilities. The employee has a right to reasonable accommodations provided by the employer to help overcome any physical limitations.

Under the spirit of ADA, employer and employees should work together to make these reasonable accommodations. Examples of reasonable accommodations for fibromyalgia workers (and all workers) in an assembly line setting might include:

1. Rotating jobs to minimize the chance of overuse syndrome or flare-ups when performing a single job all the time.

2. Rearranging work stations and providing ergonomic tools to optimize proper body mechanics and fibronomics.

3. Providing rubber mats where prolonged standing is required.

4. Allowing more frequent breaks during the work day.

5. Allowing scheduled time for stretching exercises.

6. Forming an education and preventive committee.

Once employers provide reasonable accommodations, the ADA does not give an employee special privileges. The individual with fibromyalgia still needs to perform his or her job acceptably and in a qualified manner. If an employee with fibromyalgia cannot meet the essential requirements of the job, he or she may

Back Bends:

Hands on hips, stand straight and bend backwards, Hold for three seconds

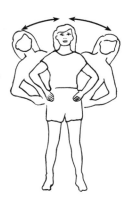

Side Bends:

Hands on hips, bend to left side, hold for three seconds, then bend to right and hold for three seconds

Overhead Reach:

Reach arms overhead as far as possible, stretch for three seconds

Wrist Stretches:

Hold hands in "prayer" position, push to the right as far as you can (you should feel stretching in your wrist tendons),hold for three seconds, repeat to the left

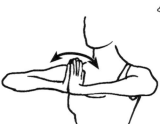
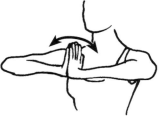

Fist Stretches:

Hold arms straight out, make fist, bend wrists in for three seconds

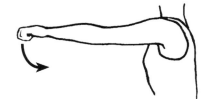

Hand Shakedown:

Arms down at sides, shake down hands for several seconds

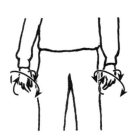

Shoulder Rolls:

Rotate shoulders around a few times

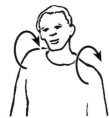

be demoted, reassigned or even terminated. There are attorneys who specialize in workplace-related issues and specifically ADA who can advise employees (and employers) on specific issues. The purpose of ADA is to give disabled people, including people with fibromyalgia, every opportunity to perform good work and make a valuable contribution to society.

In general, patients of mine who work in a small business or a professional office usually report their employer is very understanding and cooperative to accommodate the fibromyalgia issues at the work place. In larger corporations, I frequently hear from patients that an employer is not as receptive and responsive to some of the individual issues raised by workers with fibromyalgia. Know what your legal rights are under ADA and work with your union representative or legal advisor if necessary. It may be helpful to seek out other individuals with fibromyalgia or medical conditions who would benefit from reasonable accommodations at their job site so that you can all have "strength in numbers," so to speak.

The fibromyalgia worker's personal physician has an important role in helping the worker preserve gainful employment. Flare-ups of fibromyalgia occurring at work need to be evaluated by the physician and treated aggressively. Most of the time, a flare-up is related to a temporary situation that can be successfully treated and normal baseline resumed, enabling the person to return to regular job duties. Specific treatment depends on the specific area or areas of flare-up as addressed in Chapter 7.

Part of the treatment approach of a fibromyalgia worker who is experiencing a flare-up is the need to consider work restrictions which can range anywhere from complete time off work to limiting certain activities. There are various ways to restrict an individual at work, as determined by the patient and the physician.

Examples of work restrictions specific to a patient with fibromyalgia include:

1. No working more than eight hours a day, five days a week. Specifically, no overtime or weekends

2. Working part-time hours, or working day hours only, or working flexible hours

3. Avoiding temperature changes (no exposure to cold, damp weather)

4. No direct air conditioning drafts

5. No repetitive reaching or overhead use of the arms

6. No repetitive bending or leaning forward

7. No sitting, standing or walking for a certain period of time before needing to alternate between positions

In addition to work restrictions, a prescription for specific adaptive devices may be necessary. This could include:

1. Phones with headsets to minimize the reaching and bending required to manually hold the phone

2. An ergonomic chair

3. A modified typing station that includes a drop keyboard, wrist bars, and arm rests

4. A back brace to be worn at work only

In general, patients with fibromyalgia are unable to perform heavy or very heavy work. They also have a difficult time performing activities that require a lot of hand controls, or reaching and overhead use of the arms, bending and twisting, or prolonged positioning or time in one position. However, fibromyalgia patients are able to perform many activities, and can perform difficult activities as long as they have the opportunity to alternate between various positions or rotate various job activities. Many times I will place absolute restrictions on patients in terms of weight lifting (no lifting more than 20 pounds frequently and 50 pounds occasionally). If a person is experiencing a flare-up, I may temporarily place more restrictions depending on the individual situation. If the flare-up resolves and the person returns to baseline state, the restrictions can be removed. I prescribe "rest" often as part of a treatment program. If repeated flare-ups are occurring within a certain job description, it may be necessary to place permanent restrictions on the worker.

Returning to work is not a short-term goal, but a long-term one. Quite often a person can be off work, obtain therapy and treatment, and feel pretty good. But if no attempt is made to alter the job situation that caused the flare-up in the first place, it is not surprising that when the person does return to work, a flare-up occurs again. The flare-up may occur within days or may take months. The goal should not be to return to work, but to return to work and sustain work. Long-term strategies are vital in helping a fibromyalgia worker sustain gainful employment.

Most patients will indicate that their pain level is less; that is, they have a lower pain baseline whenever they are not working. The pain is not gone, but it is noticeably less. When a person returns to work, the pain baseline creeps up but hopefully will stabilize at a level that is to be considered the stable work pain baseline. Recognizing and establishing a stable work pain baseline is important for the fibromyalgia worker because sustained deviations above this baseline will constitute a flare-up and require more intensive treatment approaches.

I frequently write letters to patients' employers on behalf of the patients to explain what fibromyalgia is and how it causes muscle pain and interferes with certain activities. I will indicate the restrictions but at the same time will focus on what the person is able to do. I focus on abilities and not disabilities. Employers who are receptive to open communication between patient, doctor and employer usually make every effort to facilitate effective strategies at the work site.

The fibromyalgia worker is responsible for continuing his or her regular home program even though he or she may be working full time. If this home program is not maintained, the work pain baseline will probably creep up even higher and be very easily triggered into a flare-up or recurrent flare-up.

I frequently review the home activities and home programs of fibromyalgia patients so we can determine if there is anything that can be changed or modified so the patient hurts less at work. This ongoing review and education is a necessary part of the overall treatment program.

If various treatments such as modifying the physical stresses at work, rearranging the work station, placing work restrictions, prescribing rest, or completing a physical therapy or occupational therapy program does not help the fibromyalgia worker maintain the regular job, a different job altogether needs to be considered. Vocational counselors can help persons find different jobs within the medical restrictions, or retrain new skills, or pursue educational programs for new careers entirely. Issues of disability may need to be pursued. There are vocational bureaus at the state level that offer qualified vocational counselors.

It is my experience that the majority of fibromyalgia workers are motivated and determined to maintain their jobs and strive to maintain a stable balance between work and baseline level of pain. There are times, however, when individuals are unable to continue a certain job or any type of work due to problems associated with chronic or progressive fibromyalgia symptoms, and in these individuals the issue of disability is examined. I think that total disability should be rare in fibromyalgia, and despite all the problems, there hopefully should be something that the individual should be able to do. However, the economy is not always receptive to a worker with various restrictions due to a medical condition, and all factors have to be considered when determining whether total, partial or no disability applies to a person with fibromyalgia. The patient and doctor need to work together to reach these difficult decisions.

As a rehabilitation physician, I believe in maximizing one's abilities despite his or her medical condition. In an ideal situation, there should always be some type of job an individual with fibromyalgia could perform despite the pain. Individuals with pain who are gainfully employed will think less of their pain when performing the job. An individual with pain who is not working will have a lot more time to think about the pain. I recognize a big difference between the ideal situation and the real world, and I certainly work with each individual's situation to help the individual achieve the best possible quality of life.

The Fibromyalgia Housekeeper

11

One of the most frequent complaints given to me by patients with fibromyalgia is in the inability to perform usual housekeeping chores. The bending, reaching, lifting and pulling required of these tasks cause considerable increased pain and often lead to painful flare-ups. The fibromyalgia housekeeper is faced with the dilemma of mentally wishing to have a clean and perfect home and knowing what needs to be done, but not having the physical ability to complete the previous routine tasks, at least not being able to complete them painlessly. In reality, you only have so much energy per day and you need to determine how you are going to spend it. What does the housekeeper do?

There are some options to consider:

1. **Stop doing housework altogether.** This is usually unacceptable and the most unsanitary route to go! But daily or weekly tasks can be analyzed and determined to be acceptable if done less frequently. Consider a rotating system where different parts of the house are cleaned on different days and not done all at once. Instead of doing one heavy task in one day, spread it out into several "mini-tasks" over the course of a week.

2. **Have someone else do it, with you supervising.** This is a good way to teach responsibility to your children (or spouse) or at least this is a good way to rationalize the reason for doing this! The shared housework concept is one that can divide the responsibilities among the entire family with the fibromyalgia person doing her (or his) share of the tasks that can be comfortably handled. Some of the heavier tasks should be delegated to other family members with close supervision by the head of the household, the fibromyalgia housekeeper.

3. **Pay someone else to do it.** If you can afford it, this is the preferred method. Try to have the paid person come weekly or every other week to do the major cleaning, scrubbing and vacuuming. You can do the minor "touch-up" work in between visits.

4. **Modify the way you are doing your particular tasks.** This technique allows you to continue doing the housekeeping work, but do it in a way that is kinder to your muscles. Since housekeeping chores are done with your body in unusual and awkward positions that aggravate your fibromyalgia, proper attention must be paid to fibronomics.

Probably a combination of these options works best for each housekeeper. New strategies can be learned and used successfully.

Below is list of usual housekeeping tasks that individuals with fibromyalgia have difficulty performing.
- Running the vacuum cleaner
- Doing dishes
- Ironing
- Dusting
- Scrubbing
- Laundry
- Washing windows
- Getting objects in and out of high cupboards
- Lifting or moving heavy objects or furniture
- Prolonged writing
- Yard work of any type
- Buying, carrying and unloading groceries

Sometimes unusual projects cause flare-ups. For example, one patient described how she spent several hours decorating cakes for her boy's basketball team and experienced significant increased pain in shoulders and arms especially, from all the squeezing and reaching involved in the project. Another woman flared up her back when she was lifting heavy bird seed bags into the trunk of her car; she buys bird seed once a year. Both usual and unusual housekeeping tasks and projects can cause flare-ups in a person with fibromyalgia, so one must be constantly on guard so to speak, to try to prevent flare-ups.

The following pages are devoted to showing you some strategies and applying housekeeping fibronomics to these usual tasks. You need to find what strategy is yours.

1. Problem: Vacuuming is described as housework enemy number one, causing significant increased pain in the back, shoulders and arms.

   Fibronomics rules violated:
   Rule 1) Arms are reaching out to push and pull the heavy vacuum.
   Rule 2) Bending forward while pushing a heavy vacuum puts increased stress on the back.

   Solutions:
   (a) Obtain a lightweight vacuum cleaner to minimize the load on the arms and back.
   (b) Hold the vacuum cleaner in the following fashion: holding arms down against the side lightly holding the vacuum handle but not squeezing hard. The handle of the vacuum cleaner rests against the upper thigh and hip area. Walk forward with back maintaining a normal curvature to push the vacuum cleaner forward, and then backing up, squeeze the handle harder and pull the vacuum backwards with steady force. Repeat these steps to cover different areas of the carpet. Be sure that the arm does not reach out away from the body, but that the whole body moves forward along with the arms.

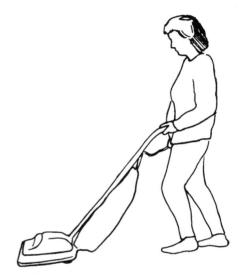

2. Problem: Nightly standing at the sink washing dishes causes severe increased back pain.

   Fibronomics rule violated:
   Rule 2) Leaning forward puts increased strain on the back.

   Solutions:
   (a) Alternate leg on a stool or inside sink cupboard to unload the back and decrease the pain.
   (b) Use paper plates, paper cups, paper cereal bowls.
   (c) Do a few dishes at a time.
   (d) If sink is too short for your height, place wash bin (plastic container) on counter top and wash from there.
   (e) Use one of those sponges that have dish detergent in the handle. This avoids using the sink at all.

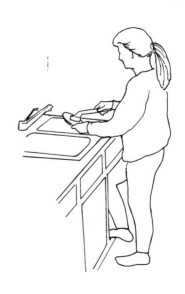

(f) Cook and eat from same dish. Use microwave bowl to cook and then eat out of it. You know, single people eat out of the pan all the time!

(g) If cooking for family, serve from stove so you don't have serving dishes and spoons to wash.

(h) If using a dishwasher, have family members load their own dishes, and assign job of unloading clean dishes to children or spouse.

3. Problem: Ironing. The bending forward and repetitive arm use cause increased pain.

Solutions:

(a) Alternate leg on a foot stool to unload the back.

(b) Avoid overextending the arm; keep elbow bent and the iron as close to the body as possible.

(c) Use a drive-through dry cleaning service.

(d) Buy fabrics that don't need ironing.

(e) Wash clothes at home; hang dry so you don't have to use dryer. Take to cleaners to press.

(f) Wear fewer clothes - wear a bathrobe!

4. Problem: Dusting. The major problem with dusting is the reaching involved to get tops of shelves and difficult areas of furniture.

Solutions:

(a) Use longer handled dust mop to allow the equipment, not your arm, to reach the spots.

(b) Use a hair dryer to blow dust off.

(c) Get rid of all knick knacks or store in glass-enclosed shelving.

5. Problem: Scrubbing. Whether scrubbing the floor, furniture or counter tops, this job is particularly difficult because of the amount of muscle force required in the actual scrubbing process. In addition to pain, muscle cramps and quick fatigue are problems.

Solution:

Use a long-handled mop when scrubbing the floor. Take advantage of any cleaning solvent that will perform the chemical scrubbing for you, so all you have to do is wipe up.

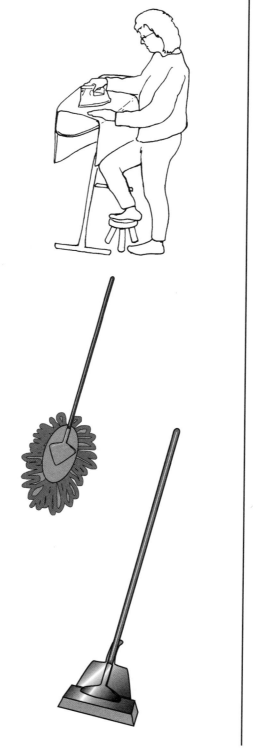

6. Problem: Doing laundry. There are various components of doing laundry that cause problems. Gathering up the dirty clothes, carrying them up and down stairs, and loading and unloading in the washer and dryer.

Solutions:
(a) Use dry cleaning services whenever possible, especially the drive-through or pick-up and delivery service.

(b) Instead of using the laundry basket to carry clothes up and down steps, place the clothes in a mesh laundry bag and throw them down the steps, or drag them up the steps behind you.

(c) Dryers that have front openings are preferred as you are able to get closer to the opening to pull out the clothes, making it easier on your low back and arms.

(d) Do one or two loads at a time - wash enough clothes for 2 or 3 days, instead of a week.

(e) Use an assistance device (a reacher-grabber device) for less bending over. You can reach into washer or dryer with it.

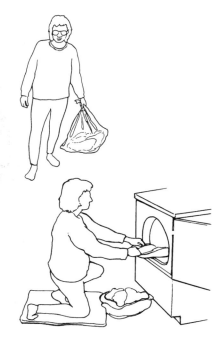

7. Problem: Washing windows. Another enemy of housekeepers and most everybody else!

Solutions:
(a) Use a long-handled window cleaner with a squeegee to clean the outside windows so you can observe proper fibronomics.

(b) Don't try to do all your windows in one day; wash only one window every other day.

(c) Hire window cleaners once a year.

(d) Close the curtains or use mini-blinds.

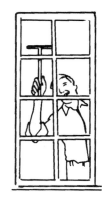

8. Problem: Getting objects in and out of high cupboards.

Solutions:
(a) Use foot stools or kitchen step ladders to bring your body higher so you can practice fibronomics when getting objects out of cupboards.

(b) Store your everyday pots and pans in your most accessible cupboards; the rarely used and heavy cooking items can go in the higher cupboards or less accessible locations.

(c) Use a reaching device.

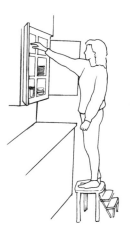

9. Problem: Lifting or moving heavy objects or furniture.

Solutions:

(a) Do not buy heavy objects unless they can be placed in their permanent resting spot.

(b) Do not lift heavy objects; leave them where they are as long as they are not bothering anything.

(c) Do not attempt to move heavy furniture during cleaning. A little dust, dirt or food particles under furniture never harmed anyone!

10. Problem: Prolonged writing. This might include check writing to pay bills, or writing letters. Writer's cramp and neck pain are very common in people with fibromyalgia.

Solutions:

(a) Instead of paying bills all at one time, designate two nights a week to write, instead of doing them all in one night.

(b) Use marker pens or pens with a medium point to minimize the amount of pressing required.

(c) Reduce the total number of checks to be written by consolidating loans or using automatic deductions.

(d) Write or type a "master" letter and Xerox copies for your different friends, adding personal tidbits to the individual's copy.

11. Problem: Yard work. This can be especially challenging since many patients with fibromyalgia love being outdoors and working on the flowers, garden, or lawn. Rather than giving this up completely, I encourage patients to find ways they can still enjoy some aspects of yard work, without doing work that is too strenuous or painful.

Solutions:

(a) Buy a garden seat and cart to allow sitting and other proper fibronomic techniques.

(b) Don't be a yard warrior. Break up large tasks into a series of smaller tasks and spread them over a longer period of time. Cut the front grass one night, the back the next and do the trimming a third night instead of doing it all in one day.

(c) Live in a condo!

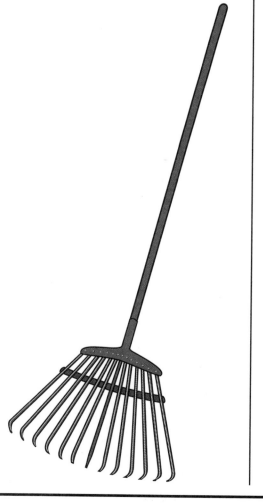

12. Problem: Grocery shopping.

Solutions:

(a) Have the grocery clerk carry your groceries out to the car and have a family member or friend carry the bags into the house.

(b) Neatly organize your grocery list by listing items according to the aisles where they are located. Always use a grocery cart (even if you just have a few groceries to buy), and use it to support your arms while you shop. Have the clerk bag the groceries "lightly."

(c) Pay a grocery helper to go out and get certain items, especially the heavier ones.

(d) Unpack some groceries at another time.

(e) Bring bags into the house but put away later.

(f) Make 2 or 3 trips a week, instead of one big haul.

(g) Shop at non-peak times. Know which stores open early or stay open late. You can park closer and avoid standing in long lines.

(h) Put laundry baskets or boxes in trunk to place grocery bags in. This way they don't slide way back in the trunk.

(i) Keep reacher-grabber in car to get items out of reach.

(j) When you go into the store, take one of those plastic baskets you can carry and put in the basket of the cart. That way you can lift more groceries from the basket out at one time; less bending and reaching is required to unload your grocery cart.

Before doing any type of house work, both physical and mental preparations are necessary. Pretend that you are about to perform an event in the "Housekeeping Olympics" and you are representing your fibromyalgia. In order to best represent your fibromyalgia for this event, you should make certain that adequate time is spent for warm up exercises that include stretching and flexibility. Emphasize the muscles that are going to be used the most and the stretches should be done just prior to the event. Mentally visualize how you will perform your event from start to finish, seeing yourself cross the finish line free from flare-up. Psych yourself up and tell yourself that you will do the best you can and that you anticipate no surprises.

Hopefully you will be successful in all your housekeeping events and win a lot of gold medals. Who knows, you may even be inducted into the Fibromyalgia Housekeepers' Hall of Fame where each recipient is honored with a bronze dust pan!

The Fibromyalgia New Mother (and New Father)   12

Fibromyalgia affects mostly women, and many of them are first bothered by symptoms in their early reproductive years, so it is very common for issues regarding pregnancy to be raised by fibromyalgia patients. This entire chapter is devoted to mothers-to-be or new mothers who have fibromyalgia.

A frequent question asked is whether or not a woman should consider getting pregnant if she has fibromyalgia. From a medical perspective there is no contraindication or unusual medical risk involved with fibromyalgia and pregnancy. Fibromyalgia itself has not been shown to cause infertility or increased miscarriages. Endometriosis frequently occurs with fibromyalgia and may cause problems with getting pregnant. Fibromyalgia seems to have a hereditary component and could be passed from mother to child, but this is not considered a dangerous medical risk or a reason to avoid pregnancy.

The main concern that the woman expresses is whether or not the pregnancy will cause a significant flare-up of her fibromyalgia, or perhaps aggravate the condition to a more severe level that persists even after the pregnancy. This fear is not unusual, nor is it without valid basis. I have treated many women in which pregnancy has played a major role in the onset of fibromyalgia. A group of women in my practice have indicated that they were never bothered by any symptoms until pregnancy, and since their first pregnancy they have had muscle pains and been diagnosed with fibromyalgia.

Another group of women have indicated that they had some pre-existing mild muscle pain, but pregnancy caused a worsening of their overall condition and led to fibromyalgia. A few individuals traced the onset of their initial low back problems and generalized fibromyalgia to their epidural procedure during the delivery. This may represent a post-traumatic fibromyalgia. Overall, a large number of women with pre-existing fibromyalgia who have been pregnant state that their condition flared up during the pregnancy; in some, the condition became worse overall, but most have said their conditions returned to their previous "stable" baseline afterwards.

Because there seem to be many people having problems with increased pain, does that mean the hopeful mother to be should be advised not to consider pregnancy because she has fibromyalgia? Absolutely not! Despite the numerous reports from these women who have been pregnant that their fibromyalgia was caused, flared up, or made worse by pregnancy, these same women will also tell you that the reward, a beautiful baby, was well worth any pain and suffering they had to endure. The benefit far outweighed the "risk." Their advice to mothers with fibromyalgia or potential mothers-to-be who question pregnancy is this: "Go ahead with it, you will be glad you did. I have no regrets and I would do the same thing all over again." I think that the more sophisticated one's knowledge is about fibromyalgia prior to the pregnancy, the better the woman will be able to anticipate and deal with any potential increased pain during the whole process of making a new family member. Of course I don't have any actual experience on pregnancy! However, the potential mother with fibromyalgia has a lot of issues to consider when deciding whether to have a child. There may already be a strained marital relationship because of the fibromyalgia, which could be further strained by adding a child to the relationship. The potential mother needs to know how much help the spouse and relatives are willing to give, especially if extra help is going to be needed because of fibromyalgia issues. Finances can be a big concern. Will the mother still be able to work and care for the baby? These issues and many more need to be carefully considered when making a decision on pregnancy.

Once a decision is made, the first thing that should be done before becoming pregnant is review all the medications that are related to fibromyalgia. A follow-up with the primary care doctor is needed to discuss the planned pregnancy and medications. Very few medications have been found to be completely safe during pregnancy; so as a rule of thumb, all prescription medicines should be reviewed with the doctor for advice on whether they can be discontinued altogether. Some medicines can be completely stopped. Others have to be weaned gradually. Remember the medicines should be completely out of her system well before the woman attempts to become pregnant. If one waits until the pregnancy is confirmed to stop the medicines, the fetus will have already been exposed to the medicine for a month. Vitamins and nutritional supplements need to be reviewed with the doctor as well prior to actual pregnancy.

Fibromyalgia dads should review their medications as well with their doctor prior to actual attempts to impregnate their partners. Sperm cells are well protected from medication side effects and the chance of causing a defective sperm that will affect the fetus at the time of conception is very remote.

Stopping medicines unfortunately can lead to increased pain, especially if medications were a crucial part of the overall pain management. There may be an initial rebound phenomenon where there is some increased pain once the body realizes the medicines are no longer in the system. However, there is also a readjustment phenomenon that occurs where the pain settles down again after it rebounded upward, and levels off to a more stable baseline, even though the baseline is possibly a little higher than the one achieved when on medications. This is the time to take advantage of more natural measures to control pain - such as using moist heating pads, hot baths, ice packs, massage, or whatever works. Certain over-the-counter pain medications may be allowed during pregnancy. Check with your primary care physician to determine which ones might be used.

A hopeful mother-to-be can take several measures to decrease the risk of fibromyalgia flare-up, whether or not medications were being used. Here are a few tips.

1. Exercise

Perform a regular exercise program that includes stretching and conditioning exercises, with emphasis on the back. This is always easier said than done, but hopefully the mother-to-be will already be performing a regular exercise program.

This program does not have to be time-consuming. Our studies have shown that performing 20 minutes of exercise three times a week will significantly improve overall conditioning and strength. Stretching exercises should be done daily however, and the trick is to integrate an overall program into your lifestyle that you will continue even after the baby is born.

2. No smoking or exposure to second-hand smoke

Nicotine decreases the blood flow to the muscles by constricting the arteries, which decreases the oxygen and increases the pain in the muscles. Cigarette smoke can also be harmful to the fetus. Frequent coughing can strain the back and cause exacerbations of the fibromyalgia.

3. Follow Fibronomics

The mother-to-be needs to perfect the techniques for proper posture and body mechanics (and fibronomics). She will really need to call upon these skills once she has the baby.

4. Get proper rest

Proper rest resets the body's physiologic mechanism to help ward off injury, illness, and stress and reduces the chance of a flare-up.

5. Schedule time for yourself

The mother-to-be should try to set aside at least an hour a day that is considered her own private time. This is the time to relax, listen to music, read a book, work on a hobby, or enjoy recreational activities. This will help deal with physical and emotional stress.

What happens to the body during pregnancy as it relates to fibromyalgia?

At the beginning of pregnancy, the body's hormones are undergoing rapid changes. The changes in the blood level concentration of various hormones such as estrogen and progesterone are necessary to enable the fetus to grow in a proper well-balanced environment and to prepare the mother for the birth. Surging hormonal changes in the first trimester can have opposite effects on the muscles of women with fibromyalgia. About half of the patients state that their muscles become more painful and they experience an overall aggravation in their fibromyalgia. In addition, many types of smells and various foods are not tolerated well, especially in the morning. These symptoms lead women to describe a feeling that they have the flu.

About half of the women, however, actually feel better from a fibromyalgia standpoint during the first trimester of pregnancy. This is somewhat surprising since normally any type of change in the body (changing hormones) usually causes increased muscle pain during pregnancy. However, not all changes must be bad, since a good percentage of women actually feel better. The reason for this improvement is probably due to hormonal changes that cause positive psychological mood changes and decreased sensitivity of the muscle pain receptors. Your body physiologically tries to make you feel "happy" during pregnancy.

During the second trimester of pregnancy, the stress to the body slowly increases. As the fetus grows, the uterus expands and the resulting protrusion shifts the body's center of gravity forward. In order to compensate for this shifting forward weight, the lumbar spine must curve backwards, and in doing so increases the swayback posture, also known as lumbar lordosis. This position creates unusual strain on the back muscles as they work harder to maintain a balanced erect posture, and the risk of back pain increases.

For every one pound of extra weight in the front of the body, there are more than two pounds of extra force exerted on the low back to compensate; so there isn't an even trade-off. The back works harder. These muscles become more fatigued and are more likely to cause pain and fatigue. Also, the back is more vulnerable to injury such as a back strain. This is true for overweight people as well.

The pregnancy hormonal changes cause the back and pelvic ligaments to soften to enable easier stretching during delivery. However this ligament softening alters the structural balance of the back, and increases the mechanical stress and results in more strain on the back.

As the pregnancy progresses, the fibromyalgia mother-to-be becomes more at risk for increased generalized pain, especially in the low back area, and increased fatigue. It is important to continue the regular stretching and conditioning exercises during pregnancy, especially for the low back.

Towards the end of pregnancy all the muscles, especially the spinal muscles are more strained. The physiologic weight gain during pregnancy has increased the energy demands and requirements of all these muscles. The extra breast weight further destabilizes the upper spine and mid-back area and contributes to unnatural strained positioning. The muscles are becoming overwhelmed and aren't "happy" anymore.

The majority of fibromyalgia women report increased muscle pain particularly in the low back towards the end of pregnancy. By then, all of the various factors have compounded to cause increased pain. It is difficult for the new mother-to-be to find comfortable positions or control her pain. I have had many of my patients participate in a supervised physical therapy program that includes heat and massage to the low back during the later stages of pregnancy for pain relief. Also, trigger point injections have been helpful. This use of this technique is not contraindicated during pregnancy, but the obstetrician and the fibromyalgia doctors need to carefully review this possible treatment method and indications for each individual patient.

Although late pregnancy may be a difficult time, it is almost the end. The mother can call upon all of her tricks and techniques to try to control the pain, with a little extra help from therapy or other medical treatments if needed, and hopefully keep the condition "manageable."

After childbirth there are additional risk factors that can cause acute exacerbation of back pain or fibromyalgia symptoms. During childbirth, sudden strenuous forces are generated through the back structures as they perform the "labor" of delivery. If the labor is prolonged, the extra long positioning and extra generated muscle forces can cause acute injury to the already vulnerable low back.

There is no evidence that natural childbirth versus epidural versus C-section makes any difference in terms of whether or not the woman will experience a flare-up of fibromyalgia back pain during childbirth. There are several fibromyalgia patients in my practice who feel that the epidural itself was the cause of the fibromyalgia, first starting off as back pain, then generalizing. It is theoretically possible that there could be a "trauma" associated with the epidural, particularly difficult epidurals as my patients described, to result in a post-traumatic fibromyalgia. However, epidurals are generally safe and only rarely result in complications, and it may be necessary and recommended for childbirth. I think the potential benefits of epidurals such as decreased pain far outweigh any potential risk of causing or flaring up fibromyalgia.

If the labor is particularly prolonged, the pregnant fibromyalgia patient should have the opportunity to shift to different positions as much as possible. Prolonged positioning is a known enemy of fibromyalgia, and if pain medications and epidurals are used, the mother-to-be will not be able to monitor pain responses as effectively to indicate when it is time to shift positions. Consequently the need to recognize and monitor prolonged positioning is important. Shifting positions can occur by moving from one side to another, alternating lying on the back with both legs straight, or with both legs bent, or with either leg bent, however the individual's labor situation will allow.

Fibromyalgia mothers become fatigued easily during labor. However, there is no evidence which shows defective uterine contraction patterns that are unique to fibromyalgia mothers, nor has there been any evidence showing that fibromyalgia mothers should have more C-sections compared to vaginal deliveries. My patients describe a longer recovery time following labor and delivery than non-fibromyalgia mothers. If the fibromyalgia mother was in labor for a long period of time, say for 48 hours, there is particular disruption of the already poor sleep cycle, more strain on the muscles and a higher potential for flare-up and delayed recovery time. The doctor needs to be aware of the mother's particular issues relating to fibromyalgia so any individual special needs can be met during the labor and delivery.

Back pain may develop within a few weeks after delivery whether it was a vaginal delivery or a C-section. The abdominal and pelvic muscles which have been stretched and weakened during the pregnancy and delivery are not able to balance the spine well. After delivery, there is decreased mobility and activity as the new mother adjusts to the post pregnancy changes and restores the body's energy supply.

Back stretching and strengthening exercises should be started within a few days after delivery, with an attempt to resume the fibromyalgia home program as quickly as possible. Sometimes extra support is needed such as a back brace or abdominal binder for a few weeks until the muscles can regain their strength and provide support. Larger breasted women who are nursing should wear a supportive bra so the extra breast weight does not further destabilize the spinal balance.

By far the biggest challenge on the new mother's fibromyalgia is the newest member of the family, the infant! This lovable, irresistible little person who weighs less than 10 pounds manages to locate him or herself into strategic positions that are most challenging to the new mother's ability to maintain proper low back and body posture. Whether the baby is in a crib, on the floor, or nestled in a car seat, the new mother must bend, and bend frequently, to a level below her waist. Twisting and reaching go hand in hand with bending, and all three of these positions are hazardous to the vulnerable back and the fibromyalgia mother. Carrying the infant is also difficult and the burden to the back increases as the child grows.

Although physical stress is a frequent cause of flare-up of pain, emotional stress can do this as well. As we know, people under stress often tense their muscles which causes spasms and pain. New mothers are certainly under a lot of stress due to the physical and emotional responsibilities of raising a newborn. Even though this type of stress may be considered "good" stress, the fibromyalgia muscles do not make the distinction between "good" and "bad" stress; they can hurt with any type of stress.

An additional imposed stress on the new mother is sleep deprivation. The sleep disorder already present with fibromyalgia is worsened by the frequent awakening of the loud and hungry infant. Lack of sleep is synonymous with being a new mother! Increased pain and fatigue result.

Mothers who breast-feed their babies are at particular risk for sleep deprivation and this is a factor to consider when deciding whether or not you want to nurse your baby. Mothers who nurse their babies will probably not be able to get back on the fibromyalgia medications as quickly as mothers who choose to bottle fed. Most of my patients choose to bottle feed, particularly after the first pregnancy because it causes fewer sleep problems and enables the partner to be more involved in the nighttime feedings.

Postpartum depression is also common, and can lead to additional poor sleep, increased fatigue, and increased pain. Given all of these stresses, it is no wonder that a new mother is more vulnerable to pain. If all of these stresses overwhelm the muscles, acute strain can occur. All of these factors can overwhelm the fibromyalgia muscles and cause a generalized flare-up.

How does the new mother decrease her risk for an acute injury or flare-up as she cares for her new baby? Here are a few tips.

1. Go back to the regular exercise program that includes stretching and conditioning exercises as soon as possible. Start with five minutes of stretching twice a day for a week and then increase ten minutes twice a day the second week. During the third week and thereafter continue with fifteen minutes a day.

   The second week after delivery begin a regular exercise program which might first include casual walking for ten minutes three to four times a week, gradually progressing to at least twenty minutes three times a week. The trick is to reintegrate a regular exercise program into your new mother lifestyle.

2. Follow Fibronomics (Moms and Dads). Although it is impossible to avoid the danger positions (bending, twisting, reaching, lifting), a new mother can learn to practice proper posture and body mechanics, specifically fibronomics, when lifting and carrying the child or engaging in other "dangerous" activities.

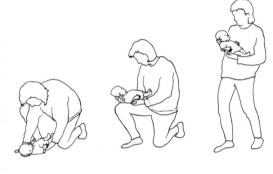

To properly place the infant on the floor, or to pick the infant up from the floor, avoid bending at the waist; instead bend at the legs and allow the legs to do the lifting while maintaining a natural back position. The one knee lift technique allows you to bring your baby close to the body before completing the lift. Keep your elbows close to your sides.

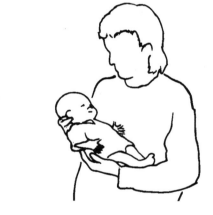

To properly carry the infant, always hold the child close to your own center of gravity which is from the chest to the naval area. Keep your elbows at your side and avoid reaching out and lifting.

To place in or pick up from the crib, first drop the crib side to the lowest position possible to minimize the bending over required. Spread your legs apart and bend your knees slightly to lower your chest and the infant as much as possible. Keep back in neutral position. Slowly bend forward with the infant still held close to your chest and then slowly open the arms, keeping your elbows against your abdomen. Set your infant down on the crib and gently ease into the proper lying position. To pick up the infant, reverse the steps.

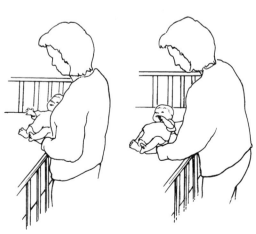

To adjust your baby's position once in the crib, try using a technique called the Golfer's Lift.

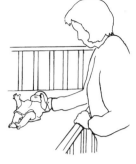

To place the infant into the car seat, put your right foot onto the car floor (if you are putting the infant onto the passenger side), and lean as close as possible to the car seat. Try to keep your elbows as close to the side as possible during the transfer into the car seat. There are swivel infant car seats available that are ideal for the fibromyalgia mother; take advantage of these special car seats to enable proper posture during car transfers.

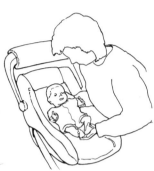

As your child gets older (and heavier), take advantage of your child's developing motor skills to protect your back. Let your child crawl onto your lap instead of picking him up. Whenever possible, sit and hold instead of stand and hold. Encourage your child to walk from point A to B instead of carrying her.

3. Get proper rest; proper sleep resets the body's physiologic mechanisms. Avoid caffeine at night. You may take naps during the day as needed.

4. Schedule your own time. Remember to set aside at least an hour a day if possible that you consider your own private time. This is when you should achieve relaxation, and do other leisurely activities such as reading a book, listening to music, working on a hobby, etc.

5. Pain relief can be obtained by various measures. Whether you are nursing or bottle feeding, check with your doctor to see what over-the-counter medications such as Tylenol, Ibuprofen, Naproxen or aspirin may be allowed. All of these medicines, except Tylenol, can help decrease both pain and any acute inflammation. (Tylenol decreases pain but does not help inflammation that occurs in a strained muscle.) Application of light heat or an ice pack can help decrease pain and spasms and increase blood flow.

Sleeping medications should usually be avoided so that the new mother can respond to the infant's needs during the night. A sleeping medicine may prevent the mother from hearing the infant cry or may have side effects such as drowsiness or confusion, or impaired balance. If the new mother is not nursing she should try to work out an on call schedule with her husband who could handle the night time feedings to allow the mother to get effective sleep, or to even use a sleeping medicine if she knew she did not have to get up at all.

If a fibromyalgia flare-up does not respond to these medicines, you would need to see your doctor for further evaluation and recommendations.

Although a new mother with fibromyalgia may be at a higher risk for developing flare-ups or acute low back strain, she can learn how to prevent or minimize these consequences so it does not interfere with the wonderful task of having and raising a new baby. Understanding the changes that occur during pregnancy and delivery that make the body more vulnerable to increased fibromyalgia pain, and taking it a few steps to improve the muscle's flexibility, strength, and overall balance, can help the new mother keep her back muscles as pain free and unnoticed as possible.

Fibromyalgia fathers need to pay careful attention to their fibromyalgia as it relates to their partner's pregnancy. The father-to-be certainly experiences a lot of stress and anxiety during the wife's/partner's pregnancy. It is natural to have concerns about the well being of the developing fetus and the mother's health, and these natural stresses can cause fibromyalgia flare-ups. In my case, being a physician father-to-be with fibromyalgia causes me to be unusually paranoid about all possible maternal and fetal complications, because I know about them. I tried to convince my wife how her pregnancies have been stressful and painful to me as well, but she didn't offer me much support in this area!

All three of my wife's pregnancies were characterized by long labors. I remember a particular disruption of the sleep cycle and a lot of fatigue, muscle pain and fogginess in thinking; and I am talking about myself too! I tried to pay proper attention to my posture as much as possible by alternating standing with sitting and pacing. I was able to fulfill my role as a supportive coach. Once the baby was born, and the baby and mother were fine, I don't remember having any pain; I was too happy.

The fibromyalgia father needs to pay special attention to proper fibronomics just like the mother does. If the mother chooses to bottle feed, as my wife did, the fibromyalgia father should be involved in the bottle feeding. I took on feeding responsibilities particularly on weekends. I am not sure which was worse, my weekend night call duties feeding the baby, or my medical on-call duties! Truthfully, I didn't mind the night feeding call duties at all because I was positively accomplishing my duty as a parent. I was able to psych myself up for these upcoming weekend duties, and my wife and I worked out an arrangement so I could catch up on my sleep when I was "off duty." This helped minimize the potential fibromyalgia complication from sleep disruption.

Even though the fibromyalgia fathers have the fibromyalgia risk with a new baby, they have it easy compared with what the mother has to go through. I know this because my wife told me so repeatedly!

Making Our Cars Fibromyalgia-Proof

13

Many of us spend considerable time in our cars every day. Commuting to and from work, running errands, traveling, and repeated trips to our doctors (!) give us the opportunity to know our car very well from the inside. We should not buy our car based on how it looks, but how functional it is for our fibromyalgia. We don't want our cars to act like us, that is, they look good on the outside, but hurt on the inside. For those of you who have the opportunity to shop around for a new car, there are some important features of the car that may help decrease your fibromyalgia pain, or help prevent it from being aggravated while you are traveling in the car.

I think an important preventive feature in a car is an adequate headrest. As you may know, the whiplash injury is one of the most common causes of post-traumatic fibromyalgia. This type of injury commonly occurs after a rear-end collision. I believe a good headrest can help reduce the severity of a whiplash injury during a rear-end collision. It does not prevent whiplash injuries, nor does it help in head-on collisions.

What happens during rear-end collision? The person sitting in a stopped care that is suddenly rear-ended will experience forward movement of the body (which acts as part of the car). The head, however, acts as an independent 10 pound object which initially stays in the same position due to inertia. The forward moving body causes the head to vigorously hyperextend or "jerk" back. The sudden hyperextension activates stretch reflexes in the front muscles of the neck which cause the head to "jerk" forward (or hyperflex) to catch up with the rest of the body. These jerking movements are the "whiplash" effects.

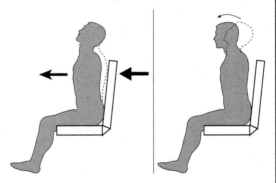

When the head and body move in opposite directions, the body quickly recognizes that this is not a good situation because the head could disconnect itself from the neck unless the body does something about it. The body reacts by tightening up the strong neck muscles in a brief protective spasm, thereby supporting the spine and head and absorbing the transmitted forces from the collision. Whereas these heroic protective efforts by the cervical, spinal, and shoulder muscles are usually successful in preventing serious neurologic injuries, injuries to the muscles and ligaments often occur.

The soft tissue injuries are the result of two events. First, the sudden force from behind causes forced extension of the neck. This stretches and tears the front and neck muscles and also causes downward pressure and compression of the structures in the back of the neck such as ligaments and joints.

Secondly, the rebound neck flexion and brief protective spasm stretches the ligaments and muscles in the back of the neck and compresses the front of the neck. The stretching that occurs on the ligaments and neck muscles causes tears and injuries and results in pain.

Different parts of the neck can be injured unequally depending on the position of the head at the time of the collision, or if the impact was not directly to the rear but more to one side or the other. Not all strains that occur from whiplash injuries ultimately result in post-traumatic fibromyalgia. Also there is usually no correlation between the severity of the rear end collision and whether or not a person develops a severe whiplash injury. The key cause of the injury is the actual "whiplash" reaction which can be triggered by any impact whether minor or major.

Is there any way to prevent a few split seconds of trauma from causing a lifetime of pain? Obviously we cannot avoid rear-end collisions, but we can try to minimize the amount of jerking back (and forward) that our head experiences during the rear-end collision by having a proper sturdy headrest. Many times the car headrest is not in the right position, is all the way down, or it is not designed well. Many of my patients who have been involved in rear-end collisions and developed post-traumatic fibromyalgia, reported that the headrest broke off during the accident. Most everyone indicates they never considered the headrest to be an important preventive device in the car. Because of my experience with so many people with whiplash injuries, I make certain that all my vehicles have an adequate headrest for the driver and all the passengers. In fact when I purchased a mini-van, my main priority was making sure that the middle seat and rear seat passengers had adequate headrests. I was very surprised that very few mini-vans met this criteria.

An adequate headrest can help prevent or minimize a whiplash-type injury. When you are seated in the car, the headrest should be able to be raised to rest just behind the middle of your head. When you move your head backwards, it should very quickly come against the headrest, that is, there should not be a lot of space between the back of your head and the headrest. Make certain that the headrest has strong supports even if it is raised into the upper position so it won't snap off in the event of a rear-end collision. Ask questions and do your research so you can make knowledgeable choices. Make sure you keep the headrest up whenever you are driving or riding. Last of all, make sure no one ever hits your car from behind!

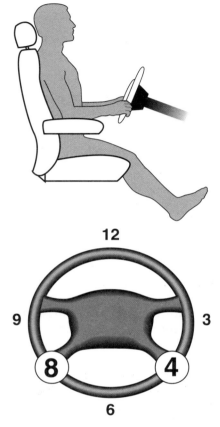

Another important car feature needed for those of us with fibromyalgia is armrests. There should be armrests on both sides of us, whether we are drivers or passengers. Prolonged driving with unsupported arms is a major cause of fatigue in our arms and upper back area. Armrests on both sides enable us to unload our upper back muscle by supporting our arms while we maintain safe control of the steering wheel. Make sure the armrests have adequate padding so as not to put pressure over the bony elbows or nerves inside the elbow. I find my arms are most comfortably positioned when the steering wheel is held in the 4 o'clock and 8 o'clock spots.

After we have taken care of our head and arms, we need to adequately support our spine. Cars should have adjustable seats and backs, particularly those with seats that move forward and backward independently of the car back movement. Power controls are better than manual devices, allowing you to make adjustments while you are driving. This feature not only enables us to find an individual comfortable position, but we are also able to adjust our positions while driving if needed. I have a favorite adjustment of my car seat, but I will change this "position" several times a week depending on whether my upper back or lower back is bothering me more. A more reclined position helps decrease my lower back pain. Each person needs to experiment in order to find the right balance of back/pelvic/leg angles. Keeping the seat as close to the steering wheel as possible helps prevent painful reaching with my arms to hold the wheel, and it also better positions my feet and bends my knee to unload my back. Some cars are equipped with lumbar supports which can be helpful if low back pain is a problem. Avoid very deep seats that you sink into, which makes it difficult to get in and out of the seats.

A good climate control system is mandatory in a car to enable us to keep our muscles at a comfortable temperature. If there is no air conditioner, we must rely on open windows for air circulation during hot days, and this invites the humidity, dust, pollen and drafts which all can irritate our sensitive skin and muscles (and mess up our perfect hair!). If you can control the air, you can keep some control of your condition. Make sure that the heating and air conditioning units are functioning properly.

The car vents should be adjusted so as to redirect the cold air away from our bodies. Direct cold air hitting our skin can trigger reflexes which cause muscle spasms and flare-ups. Warm air from defrosters can cause nausea or stuffiness if it directly hits your face, especially for those of us who are sensitive to odors and fumes and have overactive "nasal" responses from our fibromyalgia. Adjust the vents so air does not hit you directly. If certain vents cannot be adjusted to redirect the air, they can be closed.

The mirrors are also important; make sure there are lots of them so we can scan the outside world without turning our heads too far to the extremes. When we are comfortable in the driver's seat, we should be able to glance into the rear view mirror and the side mirrors by moving our eyes mostly and easily visualize everything that is happening beside and behind us. When we turn our head to the left to see our "blind spot" we should be sure that our properly positioned headrest is not obstructing the view or causing us to strain our neck too uncomfortably.

Make sure your car has an automatic drive. No stick shifts or clutches allowed unless you want your right shoulder and left leg to fall off! One patient thought a stick shift would be good exercise for her arm; she quickly learned that it caused bad flare-ups instead. Let your car do as much work for you as possible.

Once you are inside the car, you need to be careful about twisting and reaching for items that always manage to be just beyond a comfortable reach. I am talking about items that end up on the floor such as tapes, sun glasses, pens, snow scrapers, etc. One of my patients uses an assistive device called a reacher-grabber which she keeps in the front seat and uses to retrieve those impossible-to-reach items. This enables proper body mechanics. The reacher-grabber can also be used in the trunk to retrieve items and prevent the "dangerous" bending.

The Fibromyalgia Traveler

14

Vacation time should be relaxing and free from pain. However, our fibromyalgia never takes a vacation! Many of my patients complain they had more pain or a flare-up from their vacations. One particular woman was surprised at the severity of her fibromyalgia flare-up, but when I asked her exactly how she spent her vacation, she explained how she jetted to Europe, walked in five different countries in seven days, returned to the U.S. and flew across the country to California for a family reunion with many family members whom she had not seen in years. She then returned home to help her daughter move to a college dormitory for fall semester. My back started to hurt just listening to this!

Vacation time can be extremely stressful, even though this may be a happy stress. Remember, fibromyalgia does not distinguish good stress from bad stress. They both hurt just as much. There are many reasons why vacations cause paradoxical flare-ups of our fibromyalgia: Happy stress, a hectic schedule, increased physical activities (walking, hauling luggage, etc.) and distraction from our proper posture.

In our eagerness to take our vacation, we often forget about our necessary daily routine for controlling our fibromyalgia. We must remember that we are bringing our fibromyalgia with us, we have to make sure our fibromyalgia has a good time too!

Vacations, like everything else we do, have to be planned in detail. We need to try to think of everything ahead of time so that there are no surprises, and anticipate potential problems with our fibromyalgia. Always try to plan a few days at home after the vacation - strictly to rest and recover before returning to work or whatever you do in the "real world." Getting home from vacation on Sunday night and returning to work Monday morning will only invite a prolonged fibromyalgia flare-up.

So how does one prepare for vacation to include fibromyalgia? We can't fly to Europe and then see "how it goes." Trying to decide what to do after you are already there is inviting stress, confusion, disagreements and, of course, pain.

First, decide on a suitable vacation spot for both you and your fibromyalgia. Locations with hot, dry climates are best. Of course, I haven't met anyone who has taken a vacation to Siberia.

Pick locations that offer a variety of attractions or events that involve sitting as well as standing. Theme parks can be difficult places because of all the required walking and standing in lines. Avoid "locations" that require sleeping on the ground (camping out in a tent!) or sleeping on an impossible "bed," (recliner cot in an RV, Aunt Mae's sofa, etc.). My idea of camping is fishing, hiking, and boating during the day, and at night staying in an air conditioned hotel with a king-sized bed (firm mattress) and my pillows from home.

Some people have a difficult time planning for a major vacation and this stress can increase pain even before the vacation starts. I've had several patients tell me they were so overwhelmed by everything that had to be done beforehand, that they chose not to take a vacation at all.

One way to avoid being overwhelmed by the "big picture" is to plan and organize (and write down) every detail of your trip as exactly as possible, and try to follow this agenda. Take care of all your home activities such as paying the bills, doing the laundry and shopping. Prepare a list of various vacation packing duties and spread out these duties each day for two weeks before you actually leave on vacation.

By planning each day and activity, you can keep your mind occupied and off the pain as much as possible. This also breaks down the very big stressful vacation into a series of small mini-events that are not as intimidating and seem possible to accomplish and enjoy. Organizing your vacation into a series of smaller events allows you to focus your attention and energy on smaller tasks that can be accomplished, whereas if you look at the whole vacation and what you are trying to accomplish you may be overwhelmed and not feel that you have the energy or motivation to do it.

One patient plans a local getaway where she checks into a local hotel for one week a year from Monday to Friday. No one stays there during the week so it is quiet and she has the pool to herself. There is no long drive, minimal packing and expense, and lots of rest and relaxation!

Since the majority of vacationers often spend several hours more on their feet during each vacation day than they would under non-vacation circumstances, we need to recognize the potential for aggravation of our back, hip and leg symptoms because of increased walking. Carefully organize the vacation event so that you allow frequent breaks between walking, sitting and standing. It is a good idea to plan a rest day every third day for sitting and browsing only. Plan on watching a show, taking a seated sight-seeing tour, or lounging at pool side. Planned rest breaks in a hectic schedule is very much appreciated by our muscles.

If you are traveling by car, make sure you allow plenty of extra time so that you can give proper attention to your fibromyalgia. A good rule of thumb is to allow 10 extra minutes per every hour just for your fibromyalgia. Watch your position and body mechanics while you are seated in the car. Don't turn your head in an awkward position to talk to someone for long periods of time or you may develop a flare-up of your neck or shoulder muscle. Likewise, if you are taking a nap, try not to lean on a pillow in a head-tilted position for a long period of time as this can cause spasms and flare-up of the neck.

Many fibromyalgia patients are bothered by motion sickness. This is specifically aggravated in those who try to read while riding in the car. Some patients don't even attempt to take cruises because they have overwhelming motion sickness. An airplane ride is usually tolerated better except during prolonged turbulence. The apparent increased motion sickness in people with fibromyalgia probably relates to a hypersensitive vestibular system that overreacts to "extra" signals.

There are several strategies for minimizing motion sickness. If you are prone to developing motion sickness, your doctor may prescribe a motion sickness pill or patch to take with you on your vacation to use as needed. Avoid reading while riding in the car; be especially careful when looking at maps while riding in a car. When it's necessary to look at a map, look at it for no more than 15 seconds at a time before shifting your focus to outside the car at moving scenery for 15 to 30 seconds; then look at the map again, no more than 15 seconds at a time. Letting your eyes look out beyond the car enables them to relax whereas focusing on one small area while the car is moving and bouncing invites motion sickness. Breathing fresh air, getting out of the car and walking (after it has stopped, obviously!) and switching roles and becoming the driver are all helpful in combatting motion sickness.

Prolonged time spent in one position causes muscles to tighten up and become more painful. Therefore, we must take frequent position change breaks while we are traveling. Ideally, we should stop the car for every hour of driving and take a two-minute stretching break and a five-minute walking break before returning to the car and resuming driving. Every four hours we should take a five-minute stretching break, a five-minute walking break and at least a 30-minute seated break (eating a meal in a restaurant).

Watch out for drafts; vacation time seems to be a drafty time! Avoid direct air conditioning drafts in the car or in the restaurant and have a light coat to keep your arms and neck covered if it is chilly or drafty in an area. Don't roll windows down especially when driving on the freeway (or when flying!).

If you are bothered by a lot of neck pain and fatigue with prolonged driving, and feel like your head is turning into a bowling ball, and your neck a Dixie cup, you would be a good candidate to wear a soft, cervical collar during your trip. This can be helpful in allowing the neck muscles to rest while still supporting the head; it can be particularly effective while driving over bumpy areas where the jarring forces put more demands and strains on the neck muscles. I recommend that the collars should not be worn more than 50% of the time while driving or riding, and no more than one hour at a time so as not to allow the neck muscles to start stiffening up.

Help your fibromyalgia any way you can while driving or riding in a car. Taking over-the-counter pain medications 30 minutes to an hour before an anticipated strenuous activity may help dampen the pain. Rubbing our muscles with creams that generate either heat or cold can help. Bring along a tape player with ear phones and play your favorite music or relaxation tape.

If you are traveling by airplane you need to maintain proper body mechanics and frequently reposition your body. An aisle seat is the best so you can stretch out your legs and alternate your positions, especially on long flights. Take your Walkman with you. If you hate flying like I do, practice your deep breathing exercises especially just before take-off. Bring your own comfortable pillow to increase the chance of getting some restful sleep during those transcontinental or transoceanic flights at night. Your doctor may be willing to prescribe a sleep modifier to use especially on the plane to help achieve good quality sleep. In planes with larger aisleways, walk around frequently. If your budget permits, buy first class or business seats simply for the extra space. Watch out for those air blowers above you so they don't shoot cold air right onto your neck.

The luggage can be a special problem unless we take preventive measures. If you are loading your own luggage into the trunk or carrying it around for long distances, you are particularly prone to developing increased pains in your neck, shoulder, back and arm muscles. A lot of extra exertion is required to haul a closet full of clothes in three suitcases. In other words, take less! Use luggage racks, carts and wheels whenever you can. Don't sling straps over your shoulders as this will aggravate your trapezius and back muscles. The best way to transport luggage if you have fibromyalgia is to let someone else carry it for you. The next best way is to push a luggage rack on wheels in front of you. Pulling the luggage behind you is harder. If you have to carry your own luggage, make sure that you switch arms frequently, take rest stops every hundred yards where you actually set down your luggage and stretch out your arms and massage your shoulders.

Make sure you bring your own pillows with you to give yourself the best chance to get comfortable in your hotel bed or other stray bed. Many hotels have air conditioners that blow air directly on the bed area so make certain that you either block or redirect the bed air to avoid direct drafts. Have a VCR set up in your room so that you can play your favorite exercise video that you remember to bring. Always make sure that the hotel you will be staying at has a hot jacuzzi so you have a relaxing deep heat modality. Make sure you pack your bathing suit.

Don't forget to bring your medicines along, especially your sleeping pills or medicines that you use only for flare-ups in case you need them. (The medicines, not the flare-ups!) I have had patients call me from different states wondering if I could prescribe something because they forgot to bring their medicines. Never leave drugs in visible areas where they could be stolen.

There is no need to let fibromyalgia ruin a perfectly good vacation. Nor should you let it prevent you from taking a well-deserved vacation. If you remember to include fibromyalgia in your vacation preparation, you will be able to be a successful fibromyalgia traveler. Bon voyage!

Handling the Holidays

15

For many fibromyalgia patients, the worst time of the year is the holiday season, starting in late November and hitting full peak in December. This is the time of year when I see many return visits for increased fibromyalgia pain and flare-up.

There are numerous reasons why fibromyalgia is so susceptible to flaring up during the holiday season. The most prevalent reason is the increased stress that occurs at this time of the year, both positive and negative. Remember, our muscles do not know the difference between positive and negative stress; they hurt just as much with either.

The extra stresses are especially a problem for women since they are traditionally the ones responsible for preparing for the holidays. The additional responsibilities include buying gifts, wrapping, cooking, baking, decorations, and transporting various family members to and from school and social activities. All these are extra duties superimposed on the everyday responsibilities. This is a good recipe for a fibromyalgia flare-up.

Various physical stresses during the holidays include:

1. The shopping required with prolonged standing, walking, and carrying
2. The cookie baking and other cooking involved. Somehow the holiday pans are always in the highest shelves, and there seems to be some sort of relationship between the heavier the pan, the higher and more out of reach it will be.
3. The holiday decorations, putting up lights, Christmas trees, and the hundreds of other items that get arranged throughout the house and yard to prepare for the holidays
4. Increased job demands during the holidays particularly with factory workers and retailers who may work many overtime hours
5. Increased school and social activities demand more physical effort. This includes our children's school holiday plays and activities, all the holiday parties and get-togethers

In addition to physical reasons, there is increased stress caused by the weather changes. By now the weather is changing to cold and damp, particularly for those of us who live in the northern part of the country. There is less sunlight as the days get progressively shorter, and this combination disrupts our fibromyalgia baselines. Seasonal affective disorder (SAD) is a form of depression caused by lack of sunlight.

There are plenty of mental stresses during the holiday season:

1. Family relations are often strained as everyone is experiencing a higher level of stress. Numerous family get-togethers, out of town visitors staying over, and other events that brings families together for lengthy periods of time may create anticipated and actual stresses.
2. Depression is common during the holidays. Multiple factors are involved, but in fibromyalgia patients it seems that everywhere you go there is happy Christmas music and decorations, and everyone appears to be joyous, but you hurt.
3. Procrastination is a mental stress and can lead to an overwhelming sense that everything will not get done in time.
4. Worry about finances comes at this time of year with extra holiday expenses, savings depletions, tax concerns, etc.

Another cause of feeling bad around the holidays is the change in our usual eating patterns. From Thanksgiving to New Years, many of us eat large quantities of refined sugar (cookies, caramel corn, candy). We may eat out more and eat more fatty foods, gourmet foods, or unusual foods that are not a part of our routine diet. The altered eating and over-eating disrupts our usual gastrointestinal balance, and may aggravate our fibromyalgia by draining our energy, aggravating our irritable bowel symptoms, or simply causing us to not feel like ourselves.

Holidays happen at predictable times. We can recognize potential stresses and anticipate flare-ups unless we take preventive measures. Don't assume you'll get caught up in the "Holiday flare-ups" and have no control over this situation. You can take specific steps to take control of the holidays and decrease your risk of a flare-up.

Here are some tips on handling the holidays:

1. **Stress:** Don't forget to practice your stress management techniques. Recognize that this is simply a difficult time of the year, but it is only part of the year, and this stress level will not remain this high.

2. **Shopping:** Start your shopping in July. Order your gifts from catalogs instead of going out and physically shopping. First do mental shopping and know what you want to buy individuals, and then go out and buy the present you planned on buying without spending hours on your feet looking for it. If you are in the malls or stores, take frequent rest breaks and actually sit down for at least five minutes for every hour of shopping. Carefully organize your time so that you do not find yourself spending several hours of your time on your feet before your realize so much time has passed.

   Be careful about carrying packages through the store as these assorted boxes of different weights quickly multiply and become a burden to your muscles, making it difficult to follow proper fibronomics. Take advantage of any shopping carts to haul your merchandise around. Ask the stores if you can store your newly purchased items behind the counter while you finish your shopping, then gather up all the packages in one final sweep. Get two oversized shopping bags and distribute packages evenly between the bags, carrying one in each arm to better balance out the weight on your body.

   Watch out for the mall parking where the only available parking spot is practically in a different city. It is a good idea to have a non-fibromyalgia person drop you off at the mall's main entrance so you can avoid the long walking. Shop during low volume times at the stores (early morning) so you can park closer and spend less time waiting in line.

   Instead of wrapping all your gifts, take advantage of the free gift-wrapping at the stores. Use decorative gift bags or boxes that require no wrapping.

3. **Baking:** When baking or cooking, make sure that you practice your fibronomics. Instead of baking cookies, try buying cookies instead. By the time you figure the time and cost, particularly the intangible costs of increased pain/flare-up, you would be amazed that buying your cookies will be cost-effective. Make sure your kitchen work area is ergonomically efficient, that is you are not putting yourself into prolonged unnatural positions to accomplish a task. Store the pans where they can be reached easily. Have someone else get the heavy pots and pans down from the high shelves or bring them up from the basement.

   One of my patients "recycles" cookies. She puts cookies others have given her on a nice plate and takes them somewhere else! She says she doesn't need the calories!

4. **Decorating:** Spread out your decorations over a two-week period instead of trying to cram it into one day. Use ladders to put your body and arms closer to your decorations. Be creative to maintain fibronomics: place decorations at lower levels instead of up high, use decorations that wrap instead of those that need to be hung, clipped or nailed. Hire your neighbor's kid to put up your outside lights while you supervise.

   Get a smaller or miniature tree. It's a lot less work but still gives the Christmas spirit.

5. **Job:** Be particularly attentive to your job's fibronomics. If you are able to, schedule vacation time, or at least schedule a long weekend. Try to protect your weekends as much as possible so that you do not find yourself working seven days a week. If you can bring some of your work duties home to a less stressful environment, take advantage of that option.

6. **Parties:** Prioritize the parties that you must attend, and those you do not need to attend. Do not commit yourself to any party if you don't feel you will be able to attend. Learn to "just say no!" If you go to parties, try to pay attention to proper fibronomics and sit down whenever you need to. If you are unable to sit, make sure that you take breaks and if you have to, leave the party early (or go to the party fashionably late). For your own parties, try to do pot-luck instead of assuming all the responsibility. If you are able to, hire a caterer to handle your party.

7. **Dressing:** Dress warmly, making sure that the neck and hands are covered. Watch out for ice since you do not need to fall and have a contusion-related fibromyalgia flare-up. If it is icy, make sure that you have one free hand at all times to hold on to something. Wear good traction shoes or boots. Whenever there is sunlight, try to "soak it up," so to speak; sunlight can be very invigorating. Plan a vacation to a hot, dry area!

8. **Family:** Pay special attention to family stresses and family needs. Keep communication open. Schedule a private night out with your spouse for just the two of you. Take family time outs where everyone takes a break from their hectic schedules, and relaxes and communicates together.

9. **Depression:** Watch for depression. See your doctor or counselor and if you develop depression, Anti-depressant medications may be necessary. Attend support group meetings, and discuss with others problems and strategies for handling the holidays.

10. **Procrastination:** To avoid procrastination, buy a monthly planner calendar and write your necessary events, highlighting those areas, and committing only to those dates. Get together with a group of your fibromyalgia friends and plan a shopping outing in July as a group. Make a list of things that you absolutely must do and eliminate those things that are not really necessary.

11. **Financial:** Set financial limits on what you will spend during the holidays. Participate in your bank's Christmas Saver's Club to save throughout the year. Don't be tempted by such offers as "90 days, same as cash," since, if you can't afford it now, you can't afford it in 90 days. Plan how much you will spend for each gift. Be careful with your credit cards. Force yourself to commit to your savings account in the month of December, rather than depleting it.

12. **Eating:** Instead of eating large amounts of everything, eat less and have more frequent, smaller meals. Make a promise to yourself that you will not gain any weight over the holiday season. Don't neglect your exercise program since you need to burn off calories.

Don't forget to enjoy the holidays! Just because you have fibromyalgia does not automatically mean you will be miserable. You can take some active steps in preparing for the holidays and assuring that you have as much control of your fibromyalgia as possible during this difficult time.

How I Deal With My Fibromyalgia

16

I am frequently asked how I deal with my fibromyalgia. Everyone needs to find his or her own balance in life with fibromyalgia. I have developed a routine that works best for me and enables me to survive. Sometimes I don't even consider it a routine, I just get through each day. The trick is to automatically get through your day in spite of your fibromyalgia and not let the day be interrupted and essentially controlled by the fibromyalgia.

So here is my typical day:

Early in the morning I go through the process of dragging myself out of bed. I literally bribe myself and use self-motivation techniques to physically get myself out of bed. Prior to getting out I spend several minutes stretching in bed to loosen up the stiff muscles. These stretching exercises involve reaching overhead, arching, and curling the back, stretching hamstrings and legs (see stretching exercises in Physically Managing Fibromyalgia). All these stretches are done in the lying down position either on my back or on my side. After stretches, I "log roll" out of bed to minimize stress on the back. I then turn off my electric heated mattress pad.

Morning stretching is continued in the hot shower. I emphasize my worst tender areas, particularly my right trapezius, neck and mid-back regions. I prefer fairly hot water, the kind that will steam up the room, which helps prevents chills once out of the shower.

Bathroom fibronomics are practiced. I try to avoid bending over the sink so I make sure that I put my glasses on early so I can see what I'm doing from a comfortable position and not have to lean over to see in the mirror. I keep my elbows close to my side while blow-drying hair, brushing and shaving to minimize pain and fatigue in my arms and upper back. Having a shorter hair style helps save time and strain in the morning (compared to your lengthier maned women!). I also sit down in the bathroom when blow-drying hair and putting on socks to minimize back strain.

Sometimes I get sneezing spells in the morning probably from a combination of allergies, hypersensitivity to smells, and steamy air. I make certain that I assume the proper sneezing position of arms tucked tightly to the side and bent, the head and back slightly bent forward in a braced position, and knees slightly bent. In the past, I have had many flare-ups from "unprotected" sneezes; now it happens only rarely.

There is nothing unusual in the way I get dressed regarding my fibromyalgia. I prefer long-sleeved shirts even in the summer because drafts, especially from air conditioners, cause my muscles to tighten up. The usual dress shirts and ties are sufficient to cover my neck area. I wear light weight comfortable dress loafer shoes to eliminate the need to frequently bend over and tie shoes.

I have a peculiar time-saving, pain-free dressing strategy. I used to tie my ties in the morning but it was taking me entirely too long and my neck would always hurt. Being the perfectionist that I am, my tie has to be perfectly lined up, otherwise I cannot wear it. And, as all men know, you can never get it just right the first time. You may get lucky and get it right the second time, and surely by the third time it should be just right. Meanwhile, it has taken five minutes, plus, I was never able to tie my tie by looking at the mirror, so I always had to look down where I was tying. The extreme neck flexion required for me to visualize my tie caused a lot of pain. I didn't think it was right that I should start off my day already having a lot of neck pain. If I could also sleep an extra five minutes in the morning by shortening my morning routine, I was certainly in favor of that.

My solution: Once I had a tie tied perfectly, instead of taking it off completely at the end of the day, I would loosen it just enough to slip over my neck and I would hang it on the tie rack and tighten the noose up again as if it was still on my neck, but it is on the tie rack instead! When that particular tie's turn came up a few weeks later, I would simply remove it, loosen the noose again, slip it over my neck, and within seconds, I have a perfectly aligned tie.

I cannot tolerate coffee so I do not participate in the great American breakfast beverage. I usually eat a light breakfast and try to minimize my fat intake because I find that a low fat diet gives me more energy.

Fibronomics are an important aspect of my work. As a medical professional, I am supposed to use my brain instead of my body, so I can seek the positions of comfort as needed. I frequently alternate positions between sitting, standing, walking, driving, etc. When making hospital rounds, I always make certain I sit down in each patient's room and spend some time talking with the patient and examining him or her. This is good bedside manner but it also has an added benefit of unloading my back. I seek out chairs that have a good supportive back.

When I drive, I assume the proper car posture: both arms on arm rests, the usual steering wheel position of 4 o'clock, and 8 o'clock, body is close to the steering wheel as possible to eliminate reaching to the steering wheel, arms and legs bent with my knees higher than my waist. I make sure no direct air hits my body so the air conditioner vents are directed away from me. I cannot stand to drive with the windows down (especially in the Winter!)

As part of my specialty I perform a testing procedure called electrodiagnostic testing. This involves a machine that weighs approximately 35 pounds. A few times a week I must transport this machine from one office location to another, carry it up and down several flights of stairs, and put it in and out of my car. I have avoided any major flare-ups with this transport technique so far, probably because I am extremely careful with my posture.

When I actually perform these electrodiagnostic tests, I pay special attention to fibronomics because the test potentially involves a lot of reaching and bending. I make sure that I am seated. I try to have my feet up on a stool so that my knees are higher than my waist. Whenever I have to reach, I try to rest my elbow on the table, my knee or the patient, and instead of bending forward at the waist, I move my whole body forward and keep my back in a neutral position.

Whenever I am about to pick up something, bend over, reach for something or do anything involving potential strain on muscles, I pretend that this activity will cause a flare-up unless I slow down, think about what I'm about to do, and follow "perfect" body mechanics. By keeping these "unusual" activities in my conscious mind, I hope to minimize any "surprises" (flare-ups).

If I am having more pain, I have a tendency to be more fidgety, and I make a conscious effort to not appear fidgety. I may squirm a little bit in my chair or cross and uncross my legs or alternate positions more frequently.

I am always asked about the importance of maintaining proper upright sitting posture, the way our grandmothers taught us. My response to this is that I feel it is okay to slouch, because we are more comfortable that way. Sure, we hear things about how slouching is bad for our spine and posture, but when I am in the proper posture, I hurt more! Although I slouch more too, slouching becomes just as painful if I maintain any one position too long, so in the end I find myself alternating between slouching and "proper" posture. I try to find a position of comfort, rather than a position that is considered proper but painful.

I am a very time-conscious individual. All my life I have always been fully aware of what time my appointments were scheduled and I always made it a point to be early. If I am running late, I have increased anxiety. I recognize that time is an ongoing process and there is certainly a lot of it! I know I shouldn't place too much emphasis on a particular point in time on any given day. Yet, it still bothers me when I am running late.

At work, I prioritize seeing my patients at their scheduled time and giving them their allotted time. Listening to patients who have fibromyalgia and trying to help them deal with their problems takes a lot of time and I make certain that there is ample time allowed for my patients. My patients in turn come to appreciate being seen in a timely manner and feeling that they have enough time to discuss their problems.

To achieve an orderly office schedule, I see patients for scheduled appointments only, thus preventing an overwhelming number of patients coming in for a short period of time and causing quantity and quality time to be sacrificed. I certainly avoid overworking myself since I too must have ample time to recuperate so I can be effective for others. Over the years I have learned to better handle my anxieties about time and approach it like my fibromyalgia; I try to control my schedule and time as much as possible, but I expect many issues regarding time to be uncontrollable and I simply go with the flow and not get too anxious about it. Remember: *TIME HAPPENS!* I have listed some time management techniques I use.

1. Eat "fast" breakfast foods such as fruits or breakfast bars that I like and actually look forward to in the morning, so I'm motivated to get up and get going

2. Plan breakfast meetings in the morning as another way to motivate myself to get started early

3. Take "time short cuts" wherever I can, (pre-tied neck ties, wearing loafers instead of shoes with shoe-strings)

4. Try to get up at the same time and go to bed at the same time, even on weekends or days off

5. Use a day planner calendar and write down everything I am to do that involves work and social activities; keep blocks of time open for "scheduled" relaxation, especially in the evening

6. Use a car phone to make calls during prolonged stretches of driving between various work locations

7. Carry a tape recorder to dictate various business related needs whenever feasible, (in the car when I am not using the car phone)

8. Bring work home, i.e. "homework" so I am able to physically get myself into the home setting and more leisurely complete some of the business activities that do not have to be done in the office

9. Always put my keys and business notes in the same place so I don't waste time looking for them. I make a conscious effort to know exactly where I am placing these items, and if they are not in the proper location, I move them there immediately

10. Mentally plan the next day the night before

I perform frequent stretches during the day including neck and shoulder rolls and spine stretches. I do frequent door corner stretches. I try to go up and down flights of stairs instead of using the elevator, and I certainly try to do this without getting so short of breath that I can't talk.

From late afternoon to early evening, I am most at risk for fatigue. At times it can be more difficult to concentrate and my mind can feel foggy especially in the early evening. If I stay active or I am working, I don't have the problem with the fogginess that usually leads to fatigue. I have experimented with different energy pills on the market but I prefer to avoid any "stimulant-type" products.

I don't allow myself to take naps. I plan ways to stay active especially in the early evening when I am done working but before I get my second wind. I will schedule chores or run errands or do family activities. Usually by 9:00 PM I am getting my second wind, provided that I have not laid around and started "crashing" an hour earlier.

One way I try to reduce the burden of long hours at the office is to bring a lot of my work home with me. Administrative reports, dictation, and reading journals are some of the homework that I can do. Doing some of my work at home allows me to be in a more relaxed environment and makes it easier to maintain proper posture. It also gets me home earlier so that I can have quality family time and weave in the work around the family schedule. A lot of the homework occurs after I get my second wind later in the evening around 9:00 PM. I am usually in bed by 11:30 every night.

I also try to pay special attention to relaxation. There are various ways that I relax. Writing is a good form of therapy for me. I enjoy reading, movies, and just having lazy time every so often. I'm a Tetris fan also.

From an exercise standpoint, I try to practice what I preach. I perform daily stretching exercises, no matter how bad I am feeling. I do a lot of walking, both as part of my work and for recreation. I also play basketball, both leisurely and competitively. Finally, I try to maintain a regular weight-lifting program.

Okay, I don't do all of my exercises all of the time. Ideally, one should exercise every day, and at the minimum 3 times a week for a good 20 to 30 minutes. I strive for this goal, but I can honestly say I don't always accomplish it. Sometimes I justify skipping because I hurt too much or don't feel like it! I can always think of reasons why I am too busy to exercise. In the end I am comfortable with the choices I make regarding exercises and I understand that the more aggressive I am with my home program of exercising, the less pain I have. At other times I will not be as aggressive with my exercises and accept a higher baseline level of pain. I take responsibility for my own choices!

From a medication standpoint, I tend to minimize the medicines. I will take muscle nutritional supplements, ibuprofen, Tylenol, and use muscle creams. I also take a prescription sleep modifier about twice a week. If I know that I am going to have a more difficult time sleeping because of an anxiety-provoking activity that will be occurring the next day, I will allow myself to take a sleep modifier. My criteria for a sleep modifier is that it works and does not leave any sedation or hangover effect the next day. Because I take it infrequently, I have not developed a tolerance to this medicine and therefore it continues to work when I need it. I don't sleep as well when I don't take the sleeping pill, but I choose not to take the medicine every night to avoid habituation.

I certainly have flare-ups like everyone else with fibromyalgia, and I approach my flare-up like I've described. I try to identify what is causing it, and increase my treatments to try to get it under control.

The fall is the worst time of the year for me with the changing weather patterns, especially warm alternating with cold, and more humidity, combined with all of the holiday stresses. Winter is my next worse time, spring is better and summer is usually great.

In the evening I go through all my unwinding activities. I finish my homework and then try to relax with casual reading or occasionally watching TV. I make sure that I have my warm socks on and then I turn on my electric mattress pad (from fall through spring), gather up my pillows, and assume my proper fetal position. Hopefully it will be a good night!

I am not the only person in my house affected by fibromyalgia. My spouse, who does not have fibromyalgia, has to live with me. Through her support, I have been able to achieve a better level of coping with my condition. I happen to be a husband who has fibromyalgia, and she happens to be a great wife who tries to be as helpful and supportive as possible.

One of the best things about having fibromyalgia is that it forces you to examine everything in your life and prioritize things long before you would have done so otherwise. Your fibromyalgia actually gives you a head start over other people in prioritizing your time.

In the end, the single most important factor in helping me cope with my fibromyalgia is the opportunity to work with people on a daily basis who have fibromyalgia themselves. We help each other and we understand each other in our day to day struggles in dealing with fibromyalgia.

Becoming A Fibromyalgia Survivor

17

I am a fibromyalgia survivor. I have been one for over 30 years. Although my diagnosis wasn't made until my mid-20's, I can remember back as a child that I had problems which, in retrospect, were related to fibromyalgia. I had "growing pains" and many times at night I had to rub down my legs because they hurt so bad. Every time I used my arms in an outstretched position, it felt like the all energy drained out of them and I had to drop my arms. I never knew why that happened until years later when I was diagnosed with fibromyalgia. I could never comfortably ride my bike with my ram's horn handle bar because the extreme forward bending and neck extension required was too uncomfortable. My paper route caused extreme shoulder pain because of the strap supporting the bag carrying 100 papers.

As I look back, even though I didn't know about fibromyalgia, I still made some adaptations to try to eliminate and minimize whatever problem I was having at the time. In addition to massaging my legs, I would stretch my legs and my calves, walk around, use moist heat to control my "growing pains." I learned how to perform activities such as changing light bulbs, washing windows, etc. by using a step ladder and keeping my arms as close to my body as possible. I developed a technique for riding my bike where I could sit up straight and hold onto the top of the ram's horn handle bar, thus allowing my neck to be in a more neutral position. I alternated the paper bag strap on the right and left shoulder and divided my route up in half so I would only have to carry half of the papers at a time to decrease the weight on my shoulder.

I was actually becoming a fibromyalgia survivor even though I had no understanding of what fibromyalgia was. Once I was diagnosed and learned about fibromyalgia, I was able to become an active participant in my attempt to understand and manage my fibromyalgia. Education, proper posture, medication, exercises and home program are all part of taking an active role in becoming a fibromyalgia survivor.

You too can become a fibromyalgia survivor. You know what you have. You have learned strategies for managing your fibromyalgia. In my experience dealing with those with fibromyalgia, the majority of you do better and become more functional over time in spite of your painful condition. You learn strategies, both through conscious effort and practice, and some that have just "happened." You learn to appreciate a stable baseline, and when your pain worsens at times you will need to call upon all of your resources and tricks. Because you are making an effort to become a fibromyalgia survivor, I believe you will have better control over your condition as time passes. Hopefully, the flare-ups will become less frequent or less bothersome, or more quickly relieved. Hopefully, you will continue to remain functional and be able to do things you want to do. You try to make responsible decisions and lifestyle changes but maintain the highest quality of life possible.

You are not alone in your attempts to become a fibromyalgia survivor. All around you there are people in all walks of life who are struggling with the pain. You may meet some of these people and help each other out. There are many knowledgeable health professionals who can help you become a fibromyalgia survivor.

Hang in there! A lot of research is being done and we will find different medications and strategies that will help you. Some day we may even cure fibromyalgia. We don't have a cure now, but that doesn't mean that we can't do anything about it. There is a lot that can be done, and you need to do it! Good luck in becoming a fibromyalgia survivor.

The Weekly Pain Chart

How to use The Weekly Pain Chart

Insert the date under the appropriate days. For each day indicate on the pain diagram (the front and back human silhouettes) any area of bothersome pain. Indicate by placing one of the following letters: **W** for worse pain, **B** for Better or improving pain, and **S** for same or unchanged pain. To the right of the diagram is a square; place a number 1 to 10 (1 being good and 10 being terrible), depending on how you are feeling overall, in the square. Note that there is no zero as there is always some baseline pain!

In the "Causes of Worse Pain" column, briefly log in any activity or factors that you can think of that are related to your pain. This can involve activities at work, at home, stresses, weather changes, or anything else you can think of. Examples might include spending a long time driving, change in work schedule, overdoing yard work, trying a new type of exercise, standing in line for a long time, and so on.

In the last column, "Treatment," indicate what you have done for your pain. This can be anything from starting a new medicine to taking a hot shower, to modifying various types of activities. After you indicate what was done, put one of the following symbols afterwards: plus sign (+) if this treatment helped, a zero (0) if the treatment did not cause any change in the pain, and a minus sign (–) if the treatment made the pain worse.

Each day you can log in the new information. By rating and tracking your pain, and thinking about causes and trying treatments, you would be able to closely monitor your specific areas of pain and even track backwards so when a flare-up develops, you can draw some conclusions from this chart on what caused it, what is effective and what is not. Refer to Chapter 7, Managing Flare-ups, for specific details on different areas of pain/flare-up to assist you in completing the pain chart.

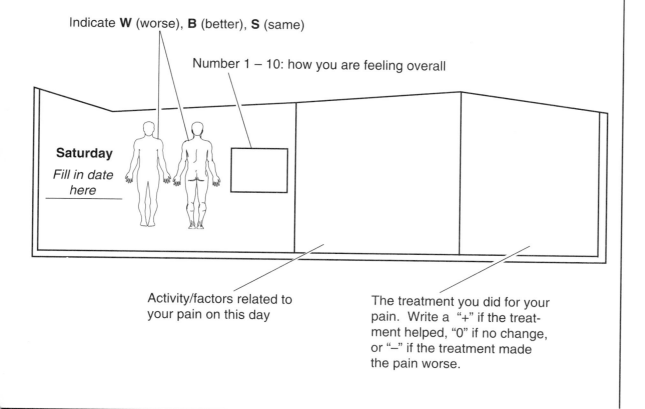

Indicate **W** (worse), **B** (better), **S** (same)

Number 1 – 10: how you are feeling overall

Saturday

Fill in date here

Activity/factors related to your pain on this day

The treatment you did for your pain. Write a "+" if the treatment helped, "0" if no change, or "–" if the treatment made the pain worse.

			Causes of Worse Pain	Treatment	Treatment: +: helped 0: no change −: made worse
Sunday _____ Indicate areas of bother- some pain on diagram W – worse B – better S – same		How am I feeling overall? 1 ——— 10 good terrible			
Monday _____					
Tuesday _____					
Wednesday _____					
Thursday _____					
Friday _____					
Saturday _____					

Index

More Books for "Helping You Live Life to the Fullest"

If you enjoyed *The Fibromyalgia Survivor,* you will be interested in other resources from Anadem Publishing. We are devoted to providing health information to assist individuals with chronic conditions in taking charge of their recovery and in getting the most out of life.

Fibromyalgia: Managing the Pain
by Mark J. Pellegrino, M.D.

Dr. Pellegrino delivers a comprehensive guide to the syndrome. It is the ideal book for the recently diagnosed FMS patient from the doctor who treats fibromyalgia patients and has it himself.

The Fibromyalgia Supporter
by Mark J. Pellegrino, M.D.

Dr. Pellegrino explains how it feels to have fibromyalgia, how you can get the support you deserve, and how you and your loved one can enjoy life together. Dr. Pellegrino combines compassion, humor and empathy with his professional expertise to provide specific steps to achieve a real "partnership" in dealing with fibromyalgia.

Understanding Post-Traumatic Fibromyalgia
by Mark J. Pellegrino, M.D.

Everyone with post-traumatic fibromyalgia will benefit from reading the first book focusing exclusively on this condition. Dr. Pellegrino presents the medical perspective on post-traumatic fibromyalgia and how it differs from other forms of fibromyalgia.

The Fibromyalgia Chef
by Mark J. Pellegrino, M.D. & Ann Evans

A new "recipe" for helping you cope with fibromyalgia. Discusses nutritional approaches to easing the symptoms of fibromyalgia, and strategies to make cooking simpler. Plus, you get over 100 easy-to-prepare recipes from Ann Evans and others with fibromyalgia.

Laugh at Your Muscles & Laugh at Your Muscles II
by Mark J. Pellegrino, M.D. & Barbara Dawkins

Two easy, light reads that you can enjoy and benefit from.

Chronic Fatigue Syndrome: Charting Your Course to Recovery
by Mary E. O'Brien, M.D.

Mary O'Brien, M.D., shares her personal experience in overcoming many of the debilitating effects of chronic fatigue syndrome. In an easy-to-read, nonmechanical format, Dr. O'Brien shares advice on treatment options and self-help steps that will help you rebuild your stamina.

TMJ — Its Many Faces
by Wesley Shankland, D.D.S., M.S.

Fibromyalgia patients frequently suffer from TMJ disorders and orofacial pain. Dr. Shankland's book is filled with step-by-step instructions on how to relieve TMJ, head, neck and facial pain.

Pills Aren't Enough
by Cody Wasner, M.D.

Pills Aren't Enough is a unique book—fictional stories of unforgettable characters help you identify your own emotions. Written by a doctor who himself has come to terms with a chronic condition, Dr. Wasner also provides you a section with thought-provoking exercises to enhance your self-discovery.

Conquering 50
by Jack J. Kleid, M.D.

In a straightforward and easy to understand way, Dr. Jack Kleid gives you the low-down on how to prevent or overcome health problems that arise after age 50. You get "pearls of wisdom," helpful hints and new and innovative strategies to help you feel and look your absolute best.

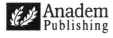 *Helping You Live Life to the Fullest*

Order Your Books Today!
— 30 Day Money Back Guarantee —

For fastest service, call 1•(800)•633-0055

Qty	Title	Price (US$)	Ohio Price*	Total
	Fibromyalgia: Managing The Pain	$12.45	$13.17	
	The Fibromyalgia Survivor	19.50	20.62	
	Understanding Post-Traumatic Fibromyalgia	16.25	17.18	
	The Fibromyalgia Supporter	15.50	16.39	
	The Fibromyalgia Chef	15.50	16.39	
	Laugh At Your Muscles	5.95	6.29	
	Laugh At Your Muscles II	5.95	6.29	
	CFS: Charting Your Course to Recovery	14.25	15.07	
	TMJ — Its Many Faces	19.50	20.62	
	Pills Aren't Enough	18.50	19.62	
	Conquering 50	$15.00	15.86	

Shipping and Handling

For 1 book, add $3.50
2–4 books, add $7.00
5–6 books, add $10
7–10 books, add $13.50
10+, please call
Priority Mail, add $2.50

*Ohio price includes 5.75% state sales tax

Subtotal _____

Add shipping and handling (see chart at left) _____

TOTAL _____

❏ Enclosed is my check, made payable to Anadem, Inc.

❏ Charge my credit card: ❏ **VISA** ❏ **MasterCard**

Card No. _____ Exp. _____

Signature _____

Name _____

Address _____

City _____ State _____ Zip _____ Phone ( ) _____

Anadem Publishing 3620 North High Street • Columbus, OH • 43214
1-800-633-0055 • FAX (614) 262-6630 • http://www.anadem.com

You can count on Anadem Publishing to keep you informed of the newest, most advanced ideas to help you get the most out of life. Let us know if you want to be placed on our mailing list to be notified of new resources. And come visit us at our website!

http://www.anadem.com